DRESS LIKE
A MILLION BUCKS
WITHOUT
SPENDING IT!

DRESS LIKE
A MILLION BUCKS
WITHOUT
SPENDING IT!

JO ANN JANSSEN
AND GWEN ELLIS

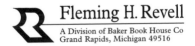

Fleming H. Revell

A Division of Baker Book House Co
Grand Rapids, Michigan 49516

© 2003 by Gwen Ellis and Jo Ann Janssen

Published by Fleming H. Revell
a division of Baker Book House Company
P.O. Box 6287, Grand Rapids, MI 49516-6287
www.bakerbooks.com

Printed in the United States of America

Library of Congress Cataloging-in-Publication Data is on file at the Library of Congress, Washington, D.C.

To

My mother, who taught me to wear it, remodel it, wear it some more, use it up, and finally use it in rag rugs. And to my beloved daddy, who left me during the writing of this book. He's no longer concerned about what to wear, because now he waits for us just inside heaven's eastern gate wearing a celestial garment.

Gwen

To

My parents, Chuck and Dorothy Pulsipher. They taught me how to make something out of nothing, figure out how to do things myself, and live a life full of love, joy, beauty, and contentment on a shoestring budget.

Jo Ann

CONTENTS

CONTENTS

INTRODUCTION

WHAT CAN YOU BUY FOR TEN BUCKS?

Whate can you buy for ten bucks? More than you ever dreamed possible, especially when it comes to clothing. I know, I know, I can hear your protests. Clothing is one of the most expensive items in a family's budget. How in the world can you save money on clothing?

That's what this book is all about. By the time you finish reading it, you will know how to save money on clothes, how to organize and repair what you have, and lots of secrets for making a few clothes work well for you. You may choose to implement all of the ideas we suggest or only a few, but even if you decide to use just one or two ideas, your budget will benefit.

In short, you can dress like a million bucks without spending it!

Recently Jo went shopping and bought a pair of Pendleton wool slacks, a Talbots sweater, and an Ann Taylor shirt—all in her colors, sizes, and styles. How much did she spend? One dollar and fifty cents! Just fifty cents per item. How, you ask? She bought them at a Salvation Army thrift store. And yes, they were all in great condition!

Think creatively! Ten dollars will buy a couple of yards of fabric. If you have or can borrow a pattern for a simple summer outfit, you can make a sundress or shorts outfit for your daughter. You can reuse buttons, trim, and zippers removed from discarded clothing to finish off the garments. Wow! That ten-dollar outfit looks great!

In this book, we'll tell you all about thrift store shopping, outlet shopping, making do, and making over. We'll tell you how to mine your own closet and how to restyle what you have to make it work better. We'll talk about basics and using accessories to get more looks. We'll talk about the fickleness of fashion and the classiness of classics. If you stick with us to the end of the book, you'll have more ideas about clothing your family on a shoestring budget than McDonald's has hamburgers. Thanks for coming along on our shoestring adventure!

ONE

LOOKIN' GOOD!

Sally Frazzle awoke one fine spring morning to the sound of birds singing and the sight of sun shining through the slats of her miniblinds. Ahhh! It was going to be a good day.

After a long and heavenly hot shower, a healthy breakfast, and the careful application of cosmetics, Sally opened her closet in search of something to wear.

The racks bulged with choices. How about the tan skirt with the coordinating jacket and blouse? That skirt hadn't fit since she gained those pounds she'd been resolving to lose for the past two years. Sally pulled out a green dress and held it up to herself in front of a full-length mirror. The shade of green gave her peachy complexion an unhealthy pall and even seemed to clash with her blond curly hair. Too bad, because the dress made her look slender and had hardly been worn. Next Sally tried on the blouse she had recently bought. Natasha looked stunning in hers, which was why Sally had run out to buy one just like it.

What looked stunning on Natasha was overwhelming on fine-boned Sally.

And so Sally's wardrobe choices ran. Too small. Needs mending. Makes hips look big. Unbecoming. Looks cheap. Too dressy. Too casual. Too loud. Too short. Outdated. Worn out. Needs a matching blouse. No shoes to go with it.

On that gorgeous spring Friday, Sally grabbed a tan dress she had dubbed "Old Faithful" because it always looked good on her. She felt confident and attractive when wearing it. She wished all her clothes fit like Old Faithful. "I think I will hit the malls this weekend and find something great on sale at Dillard's," she thought to herself as she caught a quick glimpse of her husband's dark-haired head reflected in the mirror. She hoped Ted wouldn't read her mind.

She need not have worried, because her frustrated mate was consumed with his own wardrobe dilemma. He began his clothing search by pulling out a pair of gray slacks, then remembered that the only jacket that went with them was the navy blue blazer. He always got compliments when he wore that navy blazer, but he had spilled salad dressing on it yesterday. His next choice was brown slacks and a brown tweed jacket, but the only clean, ironed shirt hanging there was a white one with faint red stripes. Not exactly a match, but it would have to do because his gray suit had been worn three times already that week and needed a good pressing. His coworkers always seemed to be so well dressed and put together—what was their secret? "Maybe," he thought to himself, "I should go shopping this weekend and see if I can fill in some wardrobe gaps. I wonder what the checkbook balance is?"

Down the hall, Ted and Sally's twelve-year-old blond daughter, Spacy, could be heard wailing, "I don't have a thing to wear!" If only her mom had bought her those designer jeans that *everyone* was wearing, she might have something she wouldn't mind being seen in. As it was, her only clean jeans ("Why doesn't Mom do laundry more often?") were so hopelessly out-of-date—she'd had them for *months*—that she was embarrassed to wear them. And *none* of her tops looked right with those jeans. Especially the tan one her mom had bought her, thinking that tan looked good on her so surely it would look good on Spacy. *Wrong!* The last possible minute before the bus came, Spacy threw on the horrid jeans and one of her brother's big T-shirts. Over it all, she pulled on a huge royal blue sweatshirt ("Thanks, Dad."). That covered most of the horror of it. As she raced out the door, she wondered if her parents would do what Amanda's mom did and let her shop with their credit card this weekend. After all, she had *nothing to wear!* Surely they would understand.

Behind Spacy lumbered her *big* big brother, Bruce. He was a throwback from a couple of generations ago when someone mixed some tall, red-haired genes into the pool. He was wearing the same pair of huge jeans he had been wearing all week. The stains from shop class went unnoticed. His shirt was clean but wrinkled from being left in the dryer too long, or perhaps he slept in it the night before—it was hard to tell which. He didn't care. He did, however, care about his sneakers. He was the only guy he knew who wasn't wearing the new Magic Marvel High-Top Springfoot Basketball Shoes. Surely his parents would want him to be playing basketball in the best shoes available so he could perform at the peak of his potential. After all, he just might get a basketball scholarship to State U. He would ask his parents tonight so he could buy the shoes tomorrow. He would find time to shop somewhere between basketball practice, mountain biking, and eating.

You have probably figured out by now that the Frazzle family needs some help with their wardrobe planning. Sally needs to discover her best colors and the fashions that are most enhancing to her figure and to her personal style. Ted could use some help creating a wardrobe in which everything goes with everything else to give him more options. Spacy and her folks need to discuss a clothing budget for her. She could also use some help in acquiring a well-organized, becoming wardrobe. It would not hurt her to learn about contentment too. And Bruce? It doesn't seem like he cares as much about his clothes as he should. Someone needs to teach him how to care for his clothing. And he needs some lessons, as does Spacy, about fighting peer pressure.

Does your family have anything in common with the Frazzles? If so, we have help for you in this book.

Getting Started

Ever since Adam and Eve first searched frantically for covering in the Garden of Eden, humans have been clothing themselves to protect themselves from weather, to keep warm, to impress others, to make a style statement, to improve appearance, and for the sake of modesty. Social pressures and personal desires can make choosing what we wear complicated and expensive.

Dressing your family can take up a big part of your budget. We should be good stewards of our resources, so it is important that we spend wisely. Your resources may be very limited. You may need to spend as little as possible on clothing to free up more cash for other things. Perhaps it just pains you to spend more than you absolutely must on anything. These are all good reasons to learn how to clothe your family on a shoestring budget. This book will teach you how.

The beautiful women in the Bible attracted kings and men of note. Now we realize the Bible doesn't mention exactly what they wore, but we are pretty sure they dressed carefully. Sure, they may have had great faces and figures, but we think they probably had learned to accentuate their best features with their choices of clothing.

We all feel much more confident and attractive when we know we look our best. Is that possible on a shoestring? It sure is! We'll teach you a few principles for looking good all the time *and* doing it on a shoestring budget. Short on money should not mean short on good looks. With our help you can learn to purchase and wear only those things that best suit you and not waste money on things that you will wear only rarely because you do not feel great in them.

Over the years we have developed some principles to guide our spending. These principles would be a great starting point for the Frazzle family. They keep us out of trouble, and they help us make wise spending decisions.

Principle #1:
Know Your Style and Stick to It.

When you follow this principle, your whole wardrobe is coordinated. Everything fits. Every garment clearly expresses who you are. You look your best in becoming fashions. How can you accomplish this miracle? Lose those pounds? No. Receive an inheritance? No. Have extensive cosmetic surgery? Nope.

The trick is discovering which colors you look best in, which fashion designs best accentuate your assets, and what your style is. Then you can determine your specific wardrobe needs based on your lifestyle.

The well-planned and well-collected wardrobe will include many pieces that coordinate with each other. If you have an idea what colors you look best in, everything you wear will enhance your natural coloring. When you own many items in the same becoming neutral color, you will have even more wardrobe flexibility.

When you know which fashion designs and clothing lines best accentuate your positive body traits and minimize your problem areas, you will buy only those things that are becoming. If you purchase things that fit correctly, you will be able to wear everything in your closet and feel comfortable and confident.

We each have a unique style, but most of our personal styles fall into one of the major style categories. When you know which style is most "you," you will not be tempted, as Sally was, to emulate someone who may look stunning but does not share your style. A classic dresser will feel more at home in her blazer and khaki slacks than in a flashy floral tent dress.

You will need to analyze the lifestyle of your family to decide what constitutes a complete wardrobe. In analyzing your family lifestyle, you should consider:

- the dress codes at places of employment
- the acceptable level of casualness or formality at your church
- where the kids attend school
- spare time activities
- your style of entertaining

Your choices may be influenced by other considerations as well, such as the climate you live in, available closet space, and how often you do laundry.

How do you decide what colors, styles, and fashion designs are best for you? There are many shoestring sources of help. We will point you in the right direction in this book.

Principle #2:
Collect the Best Quality Clothing Possible.

A shoestring buyer doesn't like to replace garments any more often than necessary. All that bargain hunting is time and energy consuming. When you buy the best quality you can afford, your clothing will look better and will wear longer and look good longer.

It doesn't cost anything to browse at expensive stores to learn what high quality clothing looks like and how it is constructed. Feel the fabrics, note the detailing, and try on clothing to see how it fits. Memorize the names of designers and brands that suit you best. Learn to recognize a high quality garment when you see one. We will show you how and where to find these high quality clothes and brand names at shoestring places and prices.

Principle #3:
Think Creatively.

You may have been frustrated for years because you can never find sleeves long enough to fit. Have you considered shopping in the men's department? Jo's daughter recently bought shorts in the boys' department—they were cheaper and they fit her better. Do you need a touch of style and color at your waist but no belt does it? Tie a scarf around your waist.

Remember Scarlett O'Hara in *Gone with the Wind*? She needed to charm some funds from Rhett Butler so she could pay the taxes on her home. She made a very stylish dress, hat, and glove ensemble from the only remaining fabric in her once grand plantation—the draperies. Rhett was no help, but her becoming outfit and flirting ways won her a husband who could pay off the taxes. We are not condoning her behavior or motives, but we do admire her creativity!

Principle #4:
Learn to Be Patient and Content.

It takes a while to build a good wardrobe. Do not compare yourself to others who have more or better clothing. Make a conscious decision to make the best of what you have. It is okay to wear the same dress to church every Sunday if that is all you can afford. Your friends will understand (if they even notice). God just wants you there.

Instead of spending what you don't have, practice patience. While you are waiting patiently to accumulate enough money to buy a suit, the suit may go on sale, you may discover a better and cheaper source of suits, or someone may give you one as a gift. You may discover that a better alternative would be a blazer and slacks. You may even decide you really need a very versatile coatdress instead! Give God time to meet your needs in his time and way. The blessings are worth it.

Principle #5:
Become a Do-It-Yourselfer.

You might have more clothes to wear if you would sew on buttons, hem up skirts, sew on patches, and fix split seams. These skills are not difficult to learn. Ask a friend to teach you, take a class, or look it up in the library. We will give you some tips on mending later in this book.

Once you learn to sew—or at least to mend—you can whip up costumes for school plays, sew simple shorts for summer fun, and even alter clothing to make it fit better.

Both of our mothers were sewers. We were brought up with the can-do attitude that enabled our parents to make the most of their modest incomes. We learned to make much of our own clothing, and today we still sew a lot. Jo frequently makes clothing for her daughter, Anna. We use our skills to keep our families' wardrobes in good shape so there is always something to wear. We keep tins of buttons handy for emergency replacements. Our needles, threads, and sewing machines are constantly on call. To keep her family trend going, Jo is training her kids to sew. They will be able to take care of themselves when they leave home. She doesn't want to do their mending forever!

Recently Jo's daughter needed a black skirt for a concert. Jo went to Goodwill. The girls' department had no black skirts, but the ladies' section had a whole rack of them. The skirts in the tiny sizes had pretty small waists. Jo bought a size 4 black skirt that looked new. Anna tried it on. It was too long and the waist needed taking in. Knowing that Anna would keep growing and would probably need another black skirt next year, Jo inserted elastic into the waistband so it fits now. Later the elastic can be removed to accommodate Anna's future growth. Next Jo hemmed the skirt with a hem deep enough to be let out next year. These alterations did not take long, and Anna had the skirt she needed for only three dollars.

Have a can-do attitude. Persevere. The feeling of accomplishment is great!

Principle #6:
Never Go into Debt to Buy Clothing.

You will have to practice patience and contentment, find creative solutions, learn to mend, and maybe even borrow a dress from a friend for a special occasion. But knowing that you did not go into debt to meet your needs is worth all the effort. Using a credit card when you do not have the cash to make a purchase means you are borrowing money. Unless you pay the entire credit card bill every month, you end up paying interest. Even the best sale prices will be negated after you add interest to your wonderful purchase price.

Special occasion clothing can break the budget if you try to purchase everything you need. You may be tempted to use that piece of plastic. But how often do you really need an evening dress with all the appropriate accessories? Is it really worth accumulating credit card debt? Jo's circle of friends has a "what's mine is yours" mentality. That means when a special occasion comes up, they share evening bags, jewelry, coats, shoes, and even dresses. Jo has lent "pearl" jewelry, basic black dress, fur coat (a family heirloom), full-length slip, evening bag, and many other things over the years. Her friends have returned them all in perfect condition along with glowing tales of special evenings. And the group of friends keeps each other out of debt.

Perhaps you can find a really sparkly evening bag like Gwen did. The tiny bag (about three inches by three inches) is studded with about two hundred rhinestones, and since these bags are so collectible, it is probably worth a small fortune. All for $0.25—that's *cents*, not dollars!

Learn to resist hype when you read ads or go shopping. We have learned that there is always another sale. There will be other opportunities to acquire the clothes you want. Trust us on this!

Neither of us has ever gone into debt to buy clothing because even if we could afford interest payments we would prefer not to pay interest on anything. Going into debt is also too scary. If we do not have an extra fifty dollars to buy something this month, how can we be sure we will have an extra fifty dollars plus interest next month to pay the Visa bill?

Both of us have had a lot of experience dressing our families on very limited budgets. Jo and her husband, Al, began their family when Al was a freelance writer. Income was very limited (How *did* we survive?) and erratic. Somehow Jo managed to clothe two little boys and, of course, herself and Al. Eventually a daughter arrived and Al got a "real" job. Working for a not-for-profit organization didn't pay a lot either, so the Janssens kept refining their shoestring lifestyle. Jo's lifestyle included entertaining Al's clients, church activities, and the bustling world of three young kids' activities.

The Janssen children are now fourteen, eighteen, and twenty. When Jo shops with them, she teaches them how to dress on a shoestring. They have picked up on her plan for accumulating basic wardrobe necessities so they always have something appropriate to wear. They know what they look good in and what their style is. They know how and where to get these needs met on a shoestring. They also know about budgeting and how much Jo is willing to spend. It makes shopping with the kids a lot more hassle free.

Gwen, like Jo, learned to dress her family on a shoestring out of necessity. Many years ago, Gwen and her husband pastored a tiny home mission church in California. When they arrived at the church, the congregation was behind in paying for most of the basic services a building needs to operate. Gwen's husband told the church members, "You will pay these bills before we take one dime from you for salary." And that is what happened. It was a long time before the salary they drew from that church could come anywhere near supporting them. One week their paycheck was thirteen dollars. Even thirty-five years ago, that was not enough for a family to survive on. Gwen's husband worked as a substitute teacher to bring in a little income. Gwen wrote articles to help out, and the other churches in the district helped to support them. It was a lean time.

In the meantime, Gwen had a growing family to keep in clothing. Since she could sew, she decided to see what fabrics she could find in thrift shops. She also begged scraps of fabrics from friends who sewed. Gwen could whip up the cutest dresses for her three-year-old daughter from little bits and pieces of fabric. She pieced and schemed until she figured out how to build a garment from less than enough fabric by making the yoke and cuffs of the tiny dresses from contrasting fabric. Sometimes she even added a contrasting band to the bottom of the dress to get the length needed. The resulting garment was often more adorable than a dress from only one fabric would have been.

One day when Gwen was in a thrift shop looking for fabrics, zippers, thread, lace, and anything else to use for sewing, she spotted a little handmade red coat, just right for her daughter. The price was three dollars. She decided right then and there that if she could buy something so cute and not even have to sew it, then maybe she needed to look around that store some more. She did and bought a yellow bunting for her soon-to-be-born baby.

Well, that set Gwen off, and she started shopping at thrift shops for what her family needed before shopping at regular retail stores. That is still pretty much her attitude today. She is known for her beautiful clothes, and any time someone comments on her wardrobe, she nearly bursts out giggling. Before writing this book, she had not let people in on her secret for dressing so well.

Because we have refined our shoestring tactics over the years and learned from our mistakes and those of our friends, we have a lot of help and encouragement for you in these pages. We are confident that you can learn to clothe your family on a shoestring. In fact, you will probably do a better job than we did because you have the benefit of our advice—much of it learned the hard way! We wish we had had this book in our hands thirty years ago! That's why the Book of Titus tells the older women (like us!) to teach the younger women how to live godly lives— you can learn from our mistakes.

But perhaps it isn't always an older-to-younger thing. A new editor recently joined Gwen's publishing team. She came from another part of the country and had no winter clothing for the cold Michigan winters. She knew about thrifting and saving money but just couldn't find the right shops. Gwen showed her the best places to find bargains. The two shop well together because their coloring is entirely different, so they never compete for the same piece of clothing. And Gwen's editor friend says she's never had so many beautiful clothes.

SHOESTRING TIPS

1. Look in the yellow pages of your local phone book under "Thrift Shops," "Secondhand Stores," and "Clothing— Consignment and Resale" to locate the shoestring sources for clothing in your area.

2. Visit those stores to get an idea of what they carry, their prices, and the overall quality of their inventory.

3. Cut up extra credit cards that tempt you to spend more than you can afford.

4. If you need help with your budget or spending habits, get it. Your church may have counseling or classes to help you. Many people have trouble with finances, so do not be embarrassed if you do as well.

5. Look in the city library or your church library for books on handling money responsibly and budgeting. We like the books written by Larry Burkett and Mary Hunt.

6. Ask God to help you be content.

7. Make friends with others in the same or a similar financial situation and encourage each other to spend wisely. Hold each other accountable. It helps to know you are not alone.

TWO

IT'S A MATTER OF STYLE

The Frazzles shared an interesting Friday evening meal. Everyone hinted at what they wanted to do on Saturday. Finally everyone admitted to wanting to go to the mall and buy clothes. The Frazzles rarely go to the mall together. The guys usually avoid the mall like the plague and the girls usually go with their friends. Uncomfortable with all this togetherness, when they arrived at the mall on Saturday they decided to split up and rendezvous in a couple of hours at the food court.

Ted approached the men's department of the first department store he came to. He nearly fled in defeat when he saw all the clothing. With so many choices, how could he possibly find what was best? He needed help. Where was Sally when he needed her? He mustered enough courage to look for the suits but passed them three times without seeing them. Finally Ted swallowed his pride and asked someone for help. As he looked through the suits, he realized he did not know his size. And there were so many colors and styles to choose from. Overwhelmed, Ted fled.

Ted reached the food court first. He carried no bags. However, once he was out of his discomfort zone, he felt his confidence returning. In the food court he made a comfortable decision: tall latte. He nursed it, hoping it would last for ninety minutes while he waited for his family.

Meanwhile, Bruce got his own taste of reality. He had no trouble finding the coveted basketball shoes. But when he saw the price tag, he knew what his parents would say. He reached the food court five minutes after his father, and they had eighty-five minutes to discuss how Bruce could come up with the money to buy those shoes.

In a dressing room at Dillard's, Sally tried on a lot of dresses. She was not sure what she wanted. Or liked. Or even what looked good on her. Trying on a black-and-white checked dress, Sally conjured up the courage to ask the salesclerk for her opinion. Salespeople often tell you that what you are trying on looks good. But luckily for Sally, this salesperson was honest. She studied Sally's face for a moment and announced: "Spring."

Huh?

The salesclerk explained that Sally has "spring" coloring and will look best in soft, warm colors. She reached into Sally's dressing room, pulled out the dresses Sally intended to try on, and went through them. She eliminated all but three.

Sally began with a cream-colored tailored coatdress. She felt very businesslike in the dress, and it looked nice on her. However, it did not excite her. Next she donned a flowery, flowing dress in tans and peaches. She felt romantic and beautiful. She didn't want to take it off, but she felt she must at least try on the last dress, a sheath in an African print. It looked nice but just wasn't her style. She put the flowery dress back on and smiled to herself. *This one is me,* she said to herself. The salesclerk told her it looked great and made the sale.

At another store, Spacy did not have her mother's good fortune. Looking at all the clothing, accessories, and jewelry, she found herself drawn to things that were unique and artsy, in bright, summery colors. But in her desire to look like everyone else, she ignored those leanings and bought a plain, mud-brown colored top just like the one on the mannequin in the junior girls' department. She priced the jeans she wanted and realized that buying them would require special parental permission.

When all four Frazzles met, only Sally felt like she had a successful shopping trip. Everyone agreed that they were overwhelmed with too many choices.

How Do We Choose?

When we go shopping, all the choices can overwhelm us. Stores display everything attractively. How do you decide what to buy? How do you know which colors look best on each person? Which fashion designs will be most becoming? What is each person's personal style? What fits the overall lifestyle of your family? Knowing these things will not only ensure wiser purchases but also narrow down the options when you shop. It will save you time, trouble, and of course money.

When Jo finally convinces her teenage son, Jonathan, that he *must* get new clothes, they know exactly what to look for. Jo will have done research to locate the best prices. Jonathan knows exactly what styles he likes. The outing is as quick and painless as possible, which makes Jonathan happier and maintains a good relationship between mother and son.

Jonathan, a "winter," looks best in white, deep blue, and black tops. His style is casual. He needs several T-shirts for school and play, a few sweatshirts for warmth, one pair of nice khakis for church, a white dress shirt, and a nice collared shirt for occasions when he needs to look nice but not dressed up. He needs two pairs of jeans and two pairs of shorts in dark blue denim. Jo and Jonathan sometimes have trouble finding pants to fit Jon's tall and extremely thin frame, but Jo has done her research and located some 28W x 32L pants. Jon still needs a belt to hold them up.

All Jon's clothes coordinate. Since he doesn't care a lot about clothes, at least Jo is comforted with the thought that his clothes go well together, fit right, look good on him, and are appropriate for all of his activities. Everyone is happy and the family stays within budget. Of course, Jonathan will grow a few more inches, so the process will have to be repeated. At least the ordeal is not too painful because Jonathan and Jo know his style. They also have a good grasp of their family's lifestyle and how it should affect each person's clothing choices. So let's talk about how a family's lifestyle influences wardrobe planning.

FAMILY LIFESTYLE

The first thing to consider when planning a wardrobe is your family's overall lifestyle. We have come up with three distinctive lifestyle categories. We are calling them "Metropolitan," "Middle American," and "Casual." You may fit precisely into one of our categories, or you may be a combination of two. Gwen is usually a Casual, but often finds herself looking like a Metropolitan when attending business meetings or speaking at conferences. Like her, your family may fit into one category most times but another at other times. Make an honest assessment so you do not buy clothes that fit some other family's lifestyle instead of your own. Be realistic. You are not the Joneses or that smartly dressed family on television. You are who you are, and your family is what it is with its own style.

The following three model families bring these styles to life. First we will look in on Dan and Sharon Metro.

The Metropolitan Lifestyle

While the Metropolitan lifestyle could be lived anywhere, Dan and Sharon Metro live in a very large city near a large lake. Since he is a broker, Dan's daily "uniform" is a nice dark suit, lightly starched white shirt with French cuffs, and well-shined wing-tip shoes. He tops it all off with a cashmere overcoat in the winter. Most of his evening outings require a similar outfit. In his spare time he may attend the opera (dark suit and tie), play golf (golf pants, shirt, athletic socks, hat, and golf shoes), or go sailing (khaki slacks or shorts, T-shirt, boater's hat). For the occasional backyard barbecue or a walk through the park, he may wear walking shorts and a golf shirt with sneakers. Dan likes to look dressed up and well groomed with his clothes pressed and starched.

While Dan is slaving away in an office, Sharon is busy attending luncheons, volunteering in the church office, and helping out in one of the kids' classrooms. She often will wear nice slacks, a simple top, blazer, and loafers. Joining Dan at formal dinners or entertaining in their home, Sharon will wear a simple black dress with pearls and high heels. Playing golf with the auction committee while planning the next auction (mothers always do at least two things at once), Sharon is comfortable but smart looking in walking shorts with matching golf shirt, hat, socks, and golf shoes.

The whole family enjoys sailing and soaking up some rays, so Sharon joins Dan on their boat wearing white shorts and a T-shirt over her swimsuit in case she decides to take a dip. She has canvas shoes on her feet and a large hat on her head for sun protection. Like Dan, Sharon always looks well dressed, freshly ironed, smart, and chic.

Both of the Metro children attend a private Christian school that requires students to wear uniforms. This makes it easy for Metro Mom, Sharon, to shop for clothing. She just has to ensure that Joe and Beth both have quality, properly-fitting sneakers and warm coats. When the Metro kids come home from school, they either go to music lessons or change into play clothes and play outside. Sometimes they have tennis or horseback riding lessons, so they need appropriate attire for those sports. Occasionally Joe and Beth help out when their parents entertain. Joe looks like a miniature Dan in his suit, white shirt, and tie. Beth elicits cries of delight from the guests when she serves hors d'oeuvres wearing a full-skirted, pink, lacy, ruffled dress. The children follow their parents' lead by always looking well dressed.

On Sunday, the whole Metro family looks their best dressed up in suits and dresses to attend the downtown Grace Community Church.

Your family may closely resemble the Metros if one of you is a professional or business executive. Perhaps you live in a community where everyone resembles the Metros. Or maybe you can relate a little better with Larry and Sue Midd.

The Middle American Lifestyle

Tucked away in a small town, quietly living their Middle American lives, are Larry and Sue Midd. Larry recently followed his dream and escaped his Dilbert-like cubicle to become the owner of his own computer business. Sue helps him run Midd Town Computer Services.

Larry's suits and ties gather dust in the back of his closet between the rare times he needs to impress a potential big client or attend a formal event like the church banquet. Most days Larry wears dress slacks with oxford button-down collar shirts and loafers. A blue blazer and a tie hang behind his office door in case he needs to dress up a bit. A tie is uncomfortable to Larry and gets in his way, and since it is *his* business he usually decides not to wear one. One of his employees always wears a dress shirt with a tie. Another employee usually shows up in jeans and a golf shirt. That's okay with Larry.

When Sue helps out in the office, she wears dress slacks in a khaki color with a knit top and a jacket. Sometimes she wears a skirt and blazer for a change. Her shoes are usually loafers or sandals.

During those rare carefree hours when the business is almost forgotten, Larry and Sue attend athletic events that their high schoolers, Luke and Annie, star in. If they have time, they might change into casual pants, turtleneck tops, and sneakers. The Midd family rarely attends functions requiring more formal attire, but Larry's best dark suit, Sue's best black dress, Luke's dress slacks, white shirt, tie, and sweater, and Annie's simple blue sheath dress suffice.

On weekends, the whole Midd family wears Bermuda or walking shorts with golf or camp-style shirts to run errands, clean house, or visit the mall. They all wear sneakers. On Sunday morning Larry wears a dress shirt and gray slacks and actually wears the blazer that usually hangs in his office. Sue has a couple of dresses and skirt-and-blouse outfits to choose from for church. The youth group is pretty casual, so Luke and Annie wear their school clothes: casual pants or jeans and collared tops. While they are not as dressy as the Metros, they would seem overdressed if they wore those clothes while visiting their cousins, the Caz family, in a California coastal town.

The Casual Lifestyle

It doesn't require a lot of closet space to accommodate Sam and Bunnie's casual wardrobes. They don't need many dresses, skirts, woven shirts, dress slacks, jackets, or suits for the Casual lifestyle. Although Sam works in an office, he isn't required to wear a suit or jacket. He puts on his tie at the last minute and removes it at 5:00 P.M. He manages to get through the workweek with a minimum number of dress slacks and shirts. During "his" time, he quickly changes into T-shirts, sneakers, and shorts or jeans. These clothes work for almost everything he does after work hours and during weekends, except when he needs a swim-suit. The coastal life is cool, and we don't mean just the weather.

Bunnie stays at home with their two toddlers, Tommy and Karen. For housekeeping, caring for the kids, meeting friends at the beach, running errands, and attending Bible study, Bun-nie wears pretty much the same clothes: shorts, a sleeveless top or T-shirt, and sandals or sneakers. Sometimes she may wear a sundress. Nothing she owns requires ironing or dry cleaning.

It doesn't take much to clothe the Caz kids. These tanned cuties wear sunsuits, shorts, T-shirts, hats for sun protection, and sometimes sneakers, if they wear any shoes at all. Usually they are barefooted.

Weekend activities center around the beach, friends, and the great outdoors. They may have a few friends over to barbecue hamburgers.

The Caz family's entire church is pretty laid-back about clothes. When he really dresses up, the pastor wears freshly ironed khaki pants, a plaid woven short-sleeved shirt, and deck shoes. For the most part, the congregation wears shorts or jeans, sleeveless shirts or T-shirts, and sandals. A few women wear nice slacks or sundresses. These people never have to buy a sepa-rate wardrobe for tropical vacations—they are living a tropical vacation!

LIFESTYLE DETERMINERS

Many things influence your family's lifestyle. Your total income may be a factor because it may limit where you live and your spare time activities. Most dressy events require high admission costs as well as the expense of dress clothes.

Your family background definitely affects who you are. That can work either for you or against you. If you were raised in a Metro home as a child, you may continue to live that way as an adult because you are comfortable with that lifestyle. On the other hand, you may consciously decide to live a different lifestyle than the one you had as a child. The lifestyle of your mate and your in-laws can also affect or change your lifestyle.

Where you work and the nature of your career may determine your lifestyle as well. A pastor's family may feel a need to live a less casual lifestyle than others because of the many social obligations they must attend. Most CEOs cannot get away with casual dress every day. On the other hand, a car mechanic would not wear an expensive suit to work.

The company you keep and the area of the country you live in will affect your lifestyle. The western United States is typically more casual than the eastern. However, your circle of friends may be the exception to that. Friends also affect your overall lifestyle.

Out in the Wild West in Colorado Springs, church attendees often wear jeans. On a hot summer day, even the pastor has been known to show up in walking shorts to preach the Saturday evening sermon. A friend's son in California has, in his twenty-some years, neither needed nor owned anything besides shorts, T-shirts, and swimsuits, plus a windbreaker for those chilly coastal winter evenings.

Taking an honest look at your current lifestyle—not the lifestyle of the Joneses, those you admire, or those you see on television—will help you buy only things that you really need. Again, you must be realistic. If you are a working mom, you may not need a lot of casual clothes. You may need workplace suits, separates, and dresses. As a stay-at-home mom, Jo needs a lot of casual clothing but very few suits and other dressy outfits because she rarely has opportunity to use them. She would like to own more but cannot justify the purchases based on her needs.

Gwen works in the office of a large Christian publisher, so her lifestyle is a little different than Jo's. Her coworkers wear what is referred to as "business casual." This seems to mean tailored slacks and skirts, loose-fitting dresses or jumpers, easy-fitting jackets, and comfortable shoes. This is a change for Gwen, who was used to wearing suits, tailored dresses, and sharp-looking jackets. Does your workplace require suits or is it more casual?

Below you will find checklists for each lifestyle. These checklists are exaggerated to make the point, and not all items under a heading will fit your family. Put check marks next to the items in all three lists that best describe you and your family. Where are most of the check marks? If they are pretty evenly divided between all three, you are probably a Middle American. You may be a mixture of two lifestyles, but most of us lean toward one category.

Metropolitan Lifestyle

__ We use our fine china and stemware on a regular basis.

__ We use our formal living and dining room often.

__ Our schedules include fancy luncheons.

__ We entertain with formal sit-down dinners.

__ Women in our family wear dresses and suits to church.

__ Men in our family wear suits or dress pants and blazers to church.

__ We attend events requiring dressy clothes several times each month.

__ We usually eat in restaurants that use linen tablecloths and napkins.

__ Our extended families are Metropolitans.

__ Our friends are Metropolitans.

__ Our children perform in fine arts programs a few times a year.

__ Husband and/or wife wears suits to work every day.

__ Kids follow strict dress codes at school or wear uniforms.

__ One of us is in the public eye often.

__ We attend opera and/or symphony concerts.

__ We attend charity events and balls.

__ Days can go by before either spouse can relax in jeans for a few hours.

__ One of us knows enough French to order intelligently at a French restaurant.

__ Wife owns and uses real pearls and diamonds.

__ Our shoes are always shined.

__ Most of our everyday clothes require dry cleaning.

__ My suspenders are held on with buttons, not clasps.

Middle American

__ We rarely use our fine china and stemware.

__ Our formal living room and dining room, if we have them, are not used very often.

__ Lunch with friends requires casual slacks.

__ We entertain with casual, potluck, family-style meals.

__ Women in our family wear dresses or skirts and blouses, or maybe even nice slacks, to church.

__ Men in our family wear dress slacks, a blazer or sweater, and maybe a tie to church.

__ We attend dressy events only a couple of times a year.

__ We usually eat in restaurants that play Muzak and use nice paper napkins and stoneware, for example Chili's or a steak house.

__ Our extended families are Middle Americans.

__ Our friends are Middle Americans.

__ Kids perform in fine arts programs two or three times a year.

__ We do presentations only occasionally.

__ Either a suit or dress slacks, jacket, shirt, and tie are worn to work by husband.

__ Wife wears slacks to work.

__ Kids wear jeans or nice slacks to school.

__ We attend sporting events and some fine arts events.

__ Best suits and dresses may go weeks unworn.

__ We own some real jewelry or nice imitations but do not use them often.

__ Only a few of our things need dry cleaning.

__ People call me by a shortened version of my given name: Bert, Beth, Sam.

__ Instead of a nice overcoat, I may wear a raincoat.

__ I had to borrow something for the New Year's Eve party at my boss's house.

The Casuals

__ If we had fine china and stemware, we would not use it.

__ If we had a formal living or dining room, it would be put to better use as a trophy room or poolroom.

__ Our schedules include meeting at the park for lunch.

__ We entertain in the backyard with our Weber grill.

__ Women in our family wear skirts, shorts, or casual slacks to church.

__ Men in our family wear jeans, shorts, or casual slacks to church.

__ We almost never attend a dressy event if we can get out of it.

__ Our favorite restaurant has ketchup and napkin dispensers on each table.

__ Our extended families are Casual.

__ Our friends are mostly Casual.

__ Our kids only perform for the occasional school program and are in sports.

__ Nobody wears a suit or dress to work unless he or she has to.

__ Our kids wear shorts, T-shirts, and jeans to school.

__ We rarely have to give presentations or do public speaking.

__ We enjoy the great outdoors often.

__ We live in jeans or shorts, T-shirts, and sneakers.

__ Our dressy clothing is rarely used.

__ We don't buy things that require dry cleaning or ironing.

__ I am known by some derivative of my given name: Bertie, Bitsy, Sammy.

__ My only pair of suspenders is red and is held on with clasps, not buttons.

__ My friends recognize me from afar because of my ever-present, distinctive baseball hat.

INDIVIDUAL STYLE

Within your overall family lifestyle, each person has a unique style. Each person's "look" or style will further narrow down the clothing choices when shopping. It will also ensure that what is purchased will actually be worn. Knowing how you want to look saves hassle and money. Al once bought Jo a very feminine, floral, lacy, and ruffled dress. She hardly ever wore it because it just wasn't her. It pays to know what your family members really want to wear, not just what you envision them wearing. (Al has decided not to buy clothing for Jo unless she is with him. No Christmas surprises there!)

There are a few major "looks" or "styles" that most of us fit into. We have divided them up into five categories that we call Sporty-Casual, Classic, Romantic, High Fashion–Dramatic, and Artsy-Creative. You may fit into one, two, or even three of them. Knowing your style or combination of styles helps make your wardrobe coordinate better and makes you feel more confident and comfortable.

Sporty-Casual

The Sporty-Casual person may show up for church in clean, comfy jeans and best golf shirt. This person likes comfortable clothes in natural fabrics. The Sporty-Casual woman wears only minimal makeup. Accessories will be simple and of natural materials like a wool muffler, leather belt, or small gold earrings. Looks and comfort may be important to the sporty-casual type, but wearing the latest trend is not. Loose or easy-fitting clothing in solids, stripes, plaids, or other simple prints are desired. Most of the clothes are easy-care cotton or wool in a variety of textures. Jo has two sons who fit this style, and Gwen is a Sporty-Casual as well.

This person doesn't fuss much with hairstyles that require a lot of time or fancy hair products. Instead, he or she will sport a simple haircut requiring no processing such as coloring or permanents.

The Sporty-Casual person wears well-worn athletic shoes, hiking boots, good-for-your-feet sandals, or loafers.

On the wouldn't-wear-it-if-you-paid-me list are ruffles, loud accessories, flowery prints, lace, trendy fashions, uncomfortable or movement-impairing styles, and anything cutesy.

This person prefers the great outdoors to being stuck indoors. Pastimes are active participation in sports and other outdoor activities. Shopping for a fashionably exciting outfit does not sound like fun.

The Classic

Jo and her husband, Al, are both Classic dressers. They have worn basically the same styles for years. Jo and Al's closet contains a few classic blazers in a few neutral colors. Jo's coordinate with her plain straight skirts, and Al's go well with his classic trousers. By choosing high quality, they make their clothes last forever. Her accessories include simple loop earrings for everyday wear, simple leather belts, the same simple shoes for dressing up, and black leather ankle-high boots to wear with slacks. Al wears classic tasseled loafers and buttoned-on suspenders with his suits, and he owns both a brown and a black belt and many classically designed ties.

The Classic person often wears his or her hair in pretty much the same style for years, making only small variations to accommodate the latest trends. These people do not fuss much with their hair. The Classic's list of wouldn't-wear-it-if-you-paid-me clothes includes anything loud, bold, trendy, or fussy. The Classic personality may enjoy sports almost as much as the Sporty-Casual type but can also be found indoors enjoying the arts. Shopping—say for new loafers—is a rare but necessary part of life.

The Romantic

Although Romantics were born in the twentieth century, their style and tastes hearken back to the 1800s. These people like to dress with style in beautiful clothing. Both manners and clothing are gracious and can be formal. Women like ruffles, lace, silk, flowery prints, very feminine looks, and fancy jewelry. Men enjoy dressing in suits, using watch fobs, and carrying walking canes.

The Romantic woman likes her long hair in curls and puts it up on her head with gentle tendrils framing her face for special occasions such as a candlelight dinner while the kids are at Grandma's.

Accessories are a favorite way to express Romantic tendencies. They may include antique jewelry or nice imitations, hats, bags, and anything that has beautiful lines and curves in it. Even their shoes will have tassels, buckles, and bows.

A true Romantic would not be caught dead wearing a plain, unadorned T-shirt, dayglow orange, or army fatigues.

The ideal vacation is a trip to Europe or a few nights in a bed-and-breakfast with days filled with shopping for antiques.

The High Fashion–Dramatic

Not just anyone can carry off the High Fashion–Dramatic style. The High Fashion–Dramatic individual enjoys putting together outfits that speak clearly of his or her strong personality. The latest trends in fashion are important—especially if they are striking in appearance. You will recognize this person right away. He or she will wear the latest hairstyle, regardless of how much work it is, regardless of whether it requires special products and processing.

This person will use bold accessories to make a style his or her own. He or she will own a vast array of interesting scarves, belts, bags, and shoes. The overall look is bold and sophisticated. There will be no frills, but there will be plenty of bright, contrasting colors and big, bold designs.

As you can imagine, a High Fashion–Dramatic would not be caught dead walking down the street in ordinary jeans and sneakers or anything passé or dowdy. Not when she could make a statement in something much more attention getting and stylish!

The High Fashion–Dramatic person would love to spend his or her vacation in a large city such as New York City, shopping for clothing by day and seeing Broadway shows at night. And he or she will look stunning while doing it.

The Artsy-Creative

Like the High Fashion–Dramatic person, the Artsy-Creative enjoys playing with clothing and accessories. However, the Artsy-Creative person isn't so concerned about what is in style this year. The adjectives "Bohemian" or "unique" often describe their wardrobes.

Many accessories and garments will be one-of-a-kind, handcrafted creations. Clothing and accessories are collected from shopping trips in art communities or created by the crafty, clever wearer. Often artists and other creative people enjoy this look and can pull it off because they know how to combine colors and prints effectively. They create the look by combining classic clothing with wide, artsy belts, hand-painted scarves, and bold or fanciful one-of-a-kind jewelry.

On their feet they may wear comfortable Birkenstocks, colorful sandals, or shoes that coordinate with their outfits.

Hairstyles may be as eye-catching as their clothing or may be simple so as not to detract from their beautiful garments. The Artsy-Creative individual enjoys spending a few days at a Shakespeare festival or participating in a craft or art fair. Shopping is for the purpose of seeing what is new in the art world and for gleaning new ideas for ways of putting things together.

At this point you may not be sure which style you are. You may conclude that you are a combination of two styles but with strong leanings toward one. Most of us cannot always wear clothing that best represents our style because not every occasion or activity lends itself to our style. A Romantic woman will not wear a flowing dress to mow the lawn. A Sporty-Casual person may have to borrow something for a formal occasion where jeans or shorts are not suitable.

Still not sure what style best fits you? See if the answers to these questions help.

1. Is there a movie or television personality you closely identify with? How does that person dress?

2. Do you know some people that you admire and want to be like? What is their style? Is it right for you?

3. What kind of clothing attracts you when you shop? What looks as if it would fit your lifestyle?

4. Which clothes in your wardrobe do you feel most at home in?

5. Do you like to dress up a lot? If not, maybe you are more Sporty-Casual.

6. Are you fashion conscious? Are you trendy? Classic or Sporty-Casual clothing may bore you.

By analyzing your family's lifestyle and each family member's personal style, you can save a lot of time, money, hassle, and even heartache by buying only what is suitable for each family member. You may now understand why some of your past purchases have hardly been worn. There are other reasons some things hang unused in your closet. In the next chapter we will look at style lines, fashion choices, and colors. We will also help you plan a well-coordinated wardrobe.

Shoestring Tips

1. Use the checklists in this chapter to determine your family's lifestyle and each family member's personal style.

2. Go through your wardrobe and remove any clothing that is not the right style for you. Is there a way you can make it your style? Can you live without it? Do you need to use it until you can replace it with something more suitable?

3. Add accessories to make plain things reflect your style.

4. Keep your eyes open for places that cater to your family's clothing style and to the styles of the individuals in your family.

5. Learn how to dress well from famous people who share your style and coloring.

6. Visit the library and peruse the fashion magazines to see the latest styles that suit you.

THREE

ACCENTUATE THE POSITIVES, ELIMINATE THE NEGATIVES

Spacy is trying on clothing in front of her full-length mirror. Nothing looks good on her today. One pair of jeans is too tight and makes her hips look too big. The brown shirt she bought yesterday makes her shoulders look too narrow, which makes her hips look too big. And the color is not becoming. Why did she buy such an ugly shirt?

She tries on a mustard yellow top that has a boat neck and horizontal stripes that makes her top half seem as big as her bottom half. But the color is ghastly on her.

A short, red sweater looks terrific, but it is warm today. A snug, sleeveless knit top only accentuates the fact that she is pear shaped. How did she end up with so many clothes and nothing to wear? "Maybe if I lost a few pounds around the hips I would look better," she says to herself. She is fooling herself. She does not need to lose weight. She will still be pear shaped no matter what she weighs. We are the way we are!

Americans are very concerned with their appearance, especially how fat they may look. We exercise, use abdomen-tightening machines, have tummy tucks, wear girdles, and try to cover or camouflage any extra pounds. Many people suffer eating disorders or go on strange diets.

God did not use a cookie cutter when he created bodies. We come in all sizes, heights, and shapes. We have short-legged people with large torsos and long-legged folks with short torsos. A few people even seem to be perfectly proportioned. Some of us have broad shoulders and little boy hips while others of us need shoulder pads to hide the fact that we have narrow shoulders and ample hips. We have mental pictures of what an ideal body looks like. Most of us will never attain that look. God made us the way we are. No amount of dieting, surgery, or clever clothing will hide the fact that we have narrow shoulders or a potbelly. Let us be content with the way God made us.

On the other hand, we do want to make the best of what we have. We shouldn't hide our assets. And it is okay to minimize our body's weak spots. There are ways to do both with the careful use of the right styles and fabrics.

Obviously, the same clothing will not best suit everyone. One man may look sleek and strong in a knit T-shirt and slacks and the next look like he's hiding a watermelon under his shirt. Besides all the usual body types, some of us have special needs that require consideration. You may be trying to hide a scar, a birth defect, one limb being significantly shorter than the other, or something else.

Once, while looking for something in a Goodwill store, Jo and her friend Karen found a pair of underwear that had been manufactured with pads sewn into the buttocks area. Since both Jo and Karen are quite adequately endowed on that particular part of their anatomies, the pads struck them as very funny. In fact, they laughed until tears streaked their faces. Then they bought the bun enhancers to use as part of a skit at a women's event at their church. Padding is one of the simple strategies for making the most of what you have—or want, as in the case of the padded underwear. We want to teach you other tricks for making the most of your assets and help you to minimize whatever you see as weak spots, as well.

HOW TO ACCENTUATE THE POSITIVE

What do you see as your best physical asset? It may be a flat tummy, a tiny waist, gorgeous legs, a long neck, or trim hips. For a guy, it may be broad shoulders or a great build. Your clothing should always draw the eye to your face and perhaps one other physical asset.

Colors are an easy way to accentuate the positive. Bright, light colors, pastels, and whites attract the eye. Using that principle, colored hose will draw the eyes to great legs. A white or pastel blouse will highlight your face. Another way to make color work for you is to use contrasting colors in accessories to catch the eye. A red belt on a pair of blue jeans looks great if your waist is slender. A colorful hair bow will make people notice a pretty head of hair.

Anything that is eye-catching or unusual accentuates the positive. Men wear flashy, colorful ties to draw attention to their faces. Prints stand out as well. A print or striped shirt will draw the eye to the chest and face. A cute hat on a child is a great device for drawing attention to an adorable face and big eyes. And a hat can hide a child's lack of hair, if need be! Artsy, one-of-a-kind accessories will also do the trick. A scarf with hand-painted cats on it, a custom-made belt in tropical hues, or a headband decorated with antique buttons will all get people's attention. Fun jewelry worn near the face for the adventurous or artsy person can bring attention to the face as well as say something about that person's interests—or simply be amusing.

Another strategy is to put shiny accessories at the place you want everyone's eyes drawn to. Gleaming metallic or jeweled earrings and necklaces draw the eye to your face. Make sure they are in correct proportion to your body—small jewelry for the small person, medium for the average-sized person, and larger for the large or tall person. A shiny belt will draw attention to a small waist. Rings, painted fingernails, and bracelets will make people notice nice hands. Colorful patent leather shoes will draw attention to small feet or great legs. Shiny hair accessories will draw attention to beautiful hair.

Some things can best be shown off by leaving them bare, within the confines of modesty and propriety, of course. Keep skirts to the knee and let your shorts be no shorter than the point where your fingertips touch your thigh when your hands dangle at your side. A pretty neck is nice to behold, but not the chest, please. If your best asset is a big bosom, ladies, this is not something you want, as a Christian, to show off. Look for another asset to feature. And men, those well-defined muscles may make you feel like Mr. Universe, but save the show for truly informal, casual, and private times. Also, guys, only bare your chest if it is truly worth showing off. Speaking of things to hide, let us now examine ways to make our nightmares go away.

Disappearing Acts

Everyone we know has something about his or her body that he or she wants to make disappear. Of course, this is not realistic, even for a magician. But we can do things to make parts visually recede. Do not emphasize your problem. Instead, lead the eye elsewhere. So if your waist goes out instead of in, you will not draw attention to this problem with a bright red, shiny belt with a big gold buckle on it. Instead, you will wear something that drapes over the waist without hugging it.

Again, color comes to our rescue. Dark, neutral colors will not draw the eye the way bright colors and whites will. Wear the same color from head to toe to create the illusion of greater height or thinness.

Avoid prints on the problem areas, as well. The busyness of prints draws attention. In fact, all the things we mentioned that would accentuate a positive should be avoided around something you wish to not draw attention to. So if you do not want anyone to notice that your hands are a manicurist's nightmare, leave the large, flashy rings in the jewelry box. Big hips will only look bigger in a loud print.

If you have bulges to hide, wear clothes that softly drape your figure and hang from your shoulders with plenty of ease down to the hem. Large people will also benefit from using the same color and vertical seams from head to toe. Draw attention toward the face. It is always a good focal point.

Some problems can best be dealt with by covering them. If you do not like your thick ankles, wear long pants and long skirts. Are your upper arms getting flabby? Avoid sleeveless tops. A birthmark on your back, an ugly scar anywhere, or dimply cellulite on your thighs never have to be viewed by the public. Keep them covered. Jo wishes hats were more popular because she has so many bad hair days.

OTHER ILLUSIONS

We have lots more tricks up our short, silk, sleek sleeves! Did you know that the fabrics you choose, the collars, and even the direction of the seams in your clothing all affect how you look? And they can all work to your advantage if you know how to use them.

Your choice of fabrics can make a body part appear bigger or smaller. Thick fabrics add bulk, so if you are fighting the battle of the bulge, do not cover the bulge in tweed. On the other hand, if your top half needs bulking up, a tweed jacket will add inches.

In short, add bulky fabrics and use layers where you need extra inches, use finer, tighter weaves and no additional layers where you want to look smaller.

Let's say you need to make your hips look smaller and your top look bigger. This is Jo's constant challenge, so she has become an expert at this. A thick sweater over a blouse with a slim skirt in summer-weight wool gabardine will help create the illusion of a better-balanced figure. A thick jacket with padded shoulders will also create the illusion of a bigger top. Jo almost always wears padded shoulders.

The opposite also works. A man with a large chest or belly will want to avoid a plaid or thick jacket. The plaid would draw attention to the largest part of his body, and the thick jacket would simply make it look bigger. He would look better in a classic blue blazer in fine wool paired with gray slacks. A bright tie will draw attention to his face. A skinny or lanky person can create the illusion of more weight by wearing bulky, full-cut clothing.

Extra fabric can also be effective in adding extra inches. Look for wide lapels and collars to make shoulders look broader. Full-cut sleeves with a little gathering at the shoulders also help. A pleated skirt without the pleats sewn down will make hips look wider. Side pockets in pants and skirts also add inches to hips. By the way, do men with full front pockets realize how funny their thighs look with all that extra bulk?

Some people try to make themselves look smaller by wearing things a size too small. A tight pair of pants only looks bad and makes people wonder if you have gained weight. A tight top on a woman simply makes her look cheap. Tight clothing is not only immodest but also shows off each dimple of cellulite, extra fold of fat, and spare tire. That is not attractive in the way you want to be attractive! Wearing things that fit correctly actually makes you look thinner and makes the clothes look like they are of high quality. You will find you are much more comfortable wearing clothing that fits properly. As we mentioned before, hide the bulges behind softly draping garments that do not accentuate the extra pounds.

The use of horizontal or vertical lines can create the illusion of better proportions. Vertical lines make you look thinner and longer. Horizontal lines make you look wider and shorter. So if you want to create the illusion of wider shoulders or a broader chest, wear shirts that have wide collars, a boat neck, horizontal stripes, or a yoke. Horizontal seams, pockets, collars, wide necklines, yokes, waistbands, cuffs, prints, and contrasting colors of all kinds may create horizontal lines.

Using these principles, if you are extremely heavy in front, you can make your chest appear smaller by avoiding front pockets and other details that draw attention or add bulk. To further diminish the appearance of your chest, wear a V neck (to add vertical lines), vertical stripes or seams, and a dull or dark color. Be sure the top is big enough to fit without allowing gaps between buttons.

Women can camouflage a waistless figure by avoiding belts, wearing longer tops that are cut or darted in at the waist, and drawing attention away from the spare tire and towards your face with jewelry or a scarf. Avoiding bulky fabrics, fullness, pockets, and bright colors can hide large hips. To trim the hips, use soft gathers, smooth fabrics, sewn down pleats, dull dark colors, and vertical seams and stripes.

OVERALL PROPORTIONS

Sometimes the only thing missing in an otherwise stunning outfit is the correct proportion. Everything else may be perfect, but if the proportions of the outfit do not work, the effect is lost.

What do we mean by proportions? Take a look in the mirror. If you are wearing jeans and a tucked in T-shirt, the T-shirt is probably about one half the length of the jeans. The ratio is one to two. This is a surefire great proportion.

Imagine your body divided into thirds: From the shoulders to the waist would be one of the thirds; from the waist to the knees would be the second of the thirds; and from the knees to the ankles would be the third of the thirds.

The best look for women is a one to two ratio, whether top to bottom or bottom to top. This explains why you see short-cropped jackets (one third) being worn with ankle-length skirts (two thirds) and long jackets (two thirds) being worn with knee-length skirts (one third). It is a nice ratio or proportion. A knee-length tunic over long pants or skirt will also give you the same one to two ratio. A thigh-length jacket over an ankle-length skirt just doesn't look right.

Study designer outfits in a fine store to learn what goes well together and to figure out how to put your own separates together most effectively. You will not only pick up on how best to put things together but also how to combine colors and texture, what is in fashion now, and how to use what you have to create today's look.

THE RIGHT COLOR

You have probably noticed that some people look absolutely stunning in certain colors. The right color enhances a person's natural coloring. If you have been told, "My, that color looks good on you," then you have received a clue as to what colors best complement your natural coloring. By only purchasing and wearing colors that are becoming, we will always look our best and feel more confident about ourselves. The added benefit is that if we only have clothes that are in becoming colors in our wardrobe, almost everything will coordinate nicely, giving us more mix-and-match options. We will need less clothing, be more satisfied, and save money.

We may not always be able to dress our kids in their best colors on a shoestring budget. While growing up, Jo, a brunette, received hand-me-downs from her older sister Sue, a blond.

What looked becoming on Sue did not look so great on Jo. That is the plight of many of our kids, and most of the time that is just fine. They grow out of clothing so quickly that we are often blessed just to have decent clothing that fits. But if you are shopping for clothing for your family, you will get more bang for your buck if you purchase things that enhance each person's natural coloring.

For example, our blond friend Kay knows she looks best in peach. She looks good in other colors, too, but peach makes her complexion glow with healthy tones. She frequently wears different shades of peach—even her warm-up suit and gardening shirt are peach. Red or royal blue washes her out. She is smart enough not to wear them. Her whole wardrobe is based on peaches, tans, and creams. Everything coordinates and she always looks great.

Which colors look best on you? If you do not know, you can do some research to find out. We have listed some books in the back of this book about color analysis, and the library may have books that cover the subject. Some cosmetic companies will do a "color draping" for you to discover not only which makeup to wear but also which colors are best for you. Amway, Mary Kay, and Avon representatives will come to you for a free consultation. Cosmetic companies with shops at the mall or counters in nice department stores have well-trained personnel who can also help you.

Few men will voluntarily visit a cosmetic counter, so they will have to try other ways to find out what they look great in. Your own family is probably a good source of advice. Finding someone else with the same color hair, skin, and eyes who always looks good can also be helpful. A wife can help by taking note of the colors and recommending them to her husband or son.

Briefly, let us give you a few color clues to help you decide on your best colors. Many consultants use the four seasons to describe color categories. We will use that strategy here.

Winter Colors

The winter person usually has very dark hair. A winter will look good in contrasting colors, deep colors, black, and white. Her best color, the one she wants close to her face because everyone says she looks so terrific in that color (and they are right!), is often black, deep red, or deep royal blue. Jo is a winter who looks best when wearing cranberry red near her face. The winter's neutral colors are black, gray, and navy blue. The winter's working wardrobe might look something like this:

A navy suit
A charcoal gray suit with skirt and pants
A red jacket
A skirt in a navy-and-gray tweed or small plaid
A camel-colored skirt
A black skirt
A deep royal blue dress
Blouse one: white
Blouse two: magenta
Blouse three: gray and navy
Blouse four: red and black
Blouse five: a sweater
Black belt and purse
Black pumps
Gray pumps
Gray-and-black tweed overcoat

Spring Colors

The spring person usually has light to medium blond hair and warm golden skin tones, with eyes quite often in the brown or gray family. Our friend Kay is a spring and looks good in tans, peach, and other muted lighter colors. Her neutral colors would be cream, tan, and golden brown. Her working wardrobe might look like this:

A tan suit with slacks and skirt
A brown suit
A cream jacket
A peach skirt
A brown-and-tan tweed or small plaid skirt
A rust skirt
A peach dress
Blouse one: cream
Blouse two: peach
Blouse three: peach and tan
Blouse four: tan and rust
Blouse five: peach and cream
Cream cardigan sweater
Brown belt and purse
Brown pumps
Cream pumps
Tan-and-brown tweed overcoat

Summer Colors

Summer colors are for those whose coloring includes blond to ash brown hair, a pink or rosy beige complexion, and bluish eyes. Gwen is a summer. Her best colors have a rose or blue undertone. Neutrals are rosy beige, taupe, and cool gray. Best colors may include rose pink, mauve, periwinkle blue, or turquoise. A summer woman's office wardrobe might look something like this:

A light bluish gray suit with skirt and slacks
A soft white (not stark white) suit
A fuchsia jacket
A gray-and-white tweed or small plaid skirt

A darker gray skirt
A dusty navy skirt
A pink dress
Blouse one: soft white
Blouse two: cool pink
Blouse three: white and dusty navy
Blouse four: fuchsia and soft white
Blouse five: pink and cool gray
Soft white cardigan
Black, dark blue, or gray belt and purse
Gray pumps
White pumps
Gray overcoat

Fall Colors

Finally the fall colors. The colors represented in fall—browns and golds—complement the fall person best. If you are a red-head, you are a fall person. Some brunettes with warm skin tones and brown eyes may also fall into this category. The fall's neutral colors include anything in the warm brown color family, rust, and olive green.

The fall woman going to the office every day might have a coordinated wardrobe that looks something like this:

A brown suit with skirt and slacks
A rust suit
Gold jacket
A tweed or small plaid skirt in browns, rusts, tans, or golds.
An olive green skirt
A tan skirt
Blouse one: cream
Blouse two: tan
Blouse three: pumpkin and rust
Blouse four: tan and rust

Blouse five: cream and olive
Brown cardigan sweater
Brown belt and purse
Brown pumps
Tan or cream pumps
Brown tweed overcoat

Now that you know your style and best colors, you can build a very coordinated wardrobe in which everything goes with everything. We hope that when you face the closet you will be able to put together a smart-looking outfit that will make you look and feel your best.

WARDROBE NEEDS

Before we go any further, you might find it helpful to make a list of the activities of each family member. Include everything: sleeping, sports, jobs (traditional dress or business casual), hobbies, lounging, working around the house, special occasions, entertaining, and other leisure activities. Next to each item, write down what clothing is needed. You will find below a long list of things to help jog your memory.

If you are lucky, your son may only require jeans and T-shirts. Most likely, though, he will require a uniform or other specialty clothing at some time. Now compare the needs to what really exists in his closets and dressers. It may be time to get rid of some excess stuff to make room for what he really needs.

During a recent spring cleaning, Jo discovered that her daughter had more dresses in her overcrowded closet than opportunities to wear them. The dresses had all been handed down from friends, so there had been no expense, but they were taking up needed closet space. Jo gave most of the dresses to another family with three little girls. Now her daughter can more easily find and retrieve what she needs from her closet.

Daily Activities

School
Job
Aerobics/exercise class
Jogging
Cleaning the house
Sports practices
Dance class
Play outside
Yard work
Hobbies
Working on the car
Playing a sport
Bible study
Night classes
Attend child's outdoor game (baseball, tennis)
Run errands
Shop
Lunch with friend
Golf
Sleeping
Watching television
Attending church

Special Events

Banquets
Speaking engagements
Dates to nice restaurants
Formal events
Semi-formal events
Musical performances

Seasonal

Seasonal parties (company Christmas party, New Year's Eve party)
Cruise
Tropical vacations
Mission trips
Vacations
Camping
Hunting
Fishing
Swimming
Snow fun
Rainy day gear
Christmas sweater or vest
Sports team uniforms and related sports gear
Sporting events

THE CORE WARDROBE

The typical family seems to go in a dozen different directions every day! And each member needs to dress correctly for each activity. It helps to have a core wardrobe that will work for 90 percent of the things you do. This core wardrobe should be a collection of well-coordinated separate pieces that mix and match with each other. By adding an accessory such as a jacket or scarf, these pieces can be transformed to work for almost any occasion. You will want to have something appropriate to wear every working day as well as for regular weekend activities like church.

BASICS FOR WOMEN

The Basic Dress

Nothing extends a wardrobe like a basic dress. A travel company sells a basic black or navy blue dress in its catalog, a pricey little number at $120. But the dress will not wrinkle when packed. It is in a loose, classic style that would look good on anyone. Here is an item that seems to be above the shoestring budget price range—but remember, this book is not about cheap; it is about *quality on a budget*. This dress will work for almost any occasion and will last for years and years. If you divide the $120 price by the number of years you should be able to wear the dress, you can figure out what the dress is actually costing you. In this case let's conservatively estimate that you could wear the dress for ten years. That's only twelve dollars per year. Not bad. Gwen recently found one of these dresses at a thrift shop. It is one of the most comfortable dresses she owns.

Gwen also bought a simple black dress at a favorite shoestring place for less than five dollars. It has short dolman sleeves and a scoop neckline, and it just skims the body. She adds a big rhinestone pin at the neckline and wears long, dangly rhinestone earrings and black hose and shoes, and the outfit looks elegant for evening. A red jacket with black buttons turns the dress into a daytime outfit.

If your basic little black dress is a two-piece outfit that looks like a dress, you have even more mix-and-match options. Your skirt can be worn with its matching top or with a lacy camisole for evening. Wear the top with any number of bottoms, from black satin trousers or trousers with a tuxedo satin strip to long swishy skirts.

Basic doesn't have to come in black or navy. Light and dark khaki, tan, cream, even burgundy or deep red can be considered basic colors. What is most important is that the basic dress be a simple, classic design, without embellishments. The embellishments will come from accessories and pieces of clothing worn over the basic dress. It's important that the dress be well constructed so that it will last for a number of years. It can have long or short sleeves depending which season it is intended for. It can be made from a number of fabrics, but lightweight wool, linen, silk, and blends that include a mixture of these fabrics and sometimes a tiny bit of polyester will last longest.

A Basic Example

For the fun of it, let's take that basic black or navy blue dress and see what we can do with it. Let's say that this basic dress is sleeveless and has a V neck.

Occasion 1: The Basic Dress at the Office

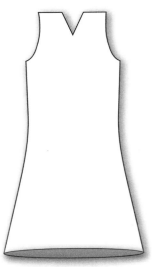

Get out the basic dress. Add a blazer jacket or a cardigan sweater, a belt, and a colorful scarf at the neckline. With classic pumps and some complementary earrings, you are ready to go to the office.

Another office look is to wear a blouse or turtleneck shirt under the dress as if it were a jumper. The dress will need to be roomy enough to accommodate a layer of clothing under it.

Occasion 2: The Basic Dress at Church

Slip on the basic dress. You can add a blazer or another more decorative jacket that has a pattern or print. Jackets can be cropped at the waist, tunic length, or anything in between. Back in vogue is a little jacket cropped well above the waist. They used to be called bolero jackets. Try one with your basic dress and see how it looks.

You can fold a big square scarf into a triangle, put it around your shoulders, and either tie it in a knot in front or fasten it with a pin in the front or at the shoulder.

You can wear a vest over your basic dress.

A silky scarf tucked into the V neck looks smart, as do beads or chains worn around your neck. Anything you put around your neck draws attention to your face—and that's a good thing.

Occasion 3: The Basic Dress on a Date

Now your basic dress really gets to put on a show. Drape a silky, filmy, or sheer scarf around your neck or shoulders. Or add lots of sparkly jewelry. Maybe a velvet or lace jacket is perfect for the occasion. Add shiny or dramatic belts. Animal prints are the rage and are very dramatic.

Tie a big silk scarf at your waist to give the dress a sarong look. Or use a long skinny silk scarf as a belt.

Make a filmy tunic to slip over your basic dress.

Accessories

Because you are not spending a lot of money on clothing, you can afford to spend some on accessory items that will truly extend your wardrobe. You may not need to spend much money on accessories as there are usually tons of them in shoestring places. People tire of their faux jewelry and don't know what to do with their silk scarves, so they toss them out. Gwen has a large collection of silk scarves picked up at just such places. She also has lots of fun earrings (some are sterling silver) purchased for pennies. Some of them are brand names found in the best department stores. Once in a while, though, you can even buy really good jewelry. She bought a pair of genuine amethyst earrings for eight dollars. She has also acquired a number of good leather handbags and belts and has yet to pay more than five dollars for any one of them.

Basic Skirt

A good quality straight or A-line skirt is essential in any woman's wardrobe. It works best if it is a neutral color and a length that is pleasing to you. Don't try to follow the latest trend in skirt length. Decide on a length that pleases you and is flattering to your legs and figure and stick to it throughout your life.

Another quality item you might want to add to your wardrobe is a good pleated skirt. It too is basic and a choice that you can wear for years.

Blazer Jacket

As a fashion statement, blazers come and go, but they are always somewhere to be seen. That's because they are so practical. A blazer in a basic color can be worn as you would a suit jacket. It can be worn for warmth like a coat. You can put a blazer over a dress or wear it with skirts, and you can even top off jeans with a blazer.

Cardigan Sweater

Here is another classic that you will wear for years if you select a good one. Wool is warm and wears well. Cotton is comfortable, but colors fade and the cotton stretches until you are often left with a baggy, shapeless mass. Acrylic and other manmade fibers pill and stretch but are easy to care for.

Back in vogue are sweater sets—a short-sleeved or sleeveless pullover and a cardigan. You might search in the back of your closet—or more likely in your mother's closet—to see if you can find a sweater set from the 1940s or 1950s. If you can, you have a real treasure. If not, you can buy new sets almost anywhere, and they are made from modern fabrics that are easy to care for.

Crew Neck Sweater

We don't know how people make their wardrobes function without a good crew neck sweater or two. Once again, crew neck sweaters can be worn with skirts, slacks, or jeans. They can be dressed up with scarves and dickeys. They can be worn over turtlenecks, shirts, and blouses. They have been around so long because they are so useful. Wool is warm, cotton is cool, and each has good points and bad points.

The good news about sweaters and jackets is that shoestring stores carry lots of them and they are very inexpensive—dare we say "cheap"?

Shoes

You don't need a lot of shoes. Women need a couple of pairs of dress pumps in basic colors—black, navy, brown, and white—a couple of pairs of flat shoes, and a pair of athletic shoes to be set for any occasion. Basic pumps can be dressed up for special occasions with inexpensive buckles and bows found in most shoe stores.

Everyone needs athletic shoes. Many of us wear them as much as we can because they are so comfortable and good for our feet. Athletes may need specialty shoes designed specifically for their sports.

Pants

You will need a couple of pairs of well-made, classic-styled pants in a straight leg. Add a couple pairs of jeans that fit well and one or two pairs of shorts of a moderate leg length.

BASICS FOR THE GUYS

Many guys are very much into basic clothing—so much so that their wardrobes can become basically boring. Their standard uniforms are suits or slacks and blazers varied with shirts and ties of various colors and combinations. The difference between a guy's wardrobe that is interesting and one that is blah is often as simple as the selection of ties and shirts he puts with the blazer and pants.

Many men require at least one suit for work or dressy occasions. A gray pinstripe will take a man to weddings, funerals, banquets, and church.

A well-made, well-fitted blazer jacket is a good investment. It will look good and keep its shape until it is worn out. It should be a neutral color that complements the wearer. Slacks should also be well made and professionally fitted. When purchasing clothing, men do well to buy at least two pairs of pants for each blazer. Jackets will far outlast slacks.

Dress shirts and ties should coordinate. Store personnel are more than happy to help with this task. Think about socks and shoes too. Shoes should be of well-constructed leather. Men should determine the length of sock they prefer and buy several pairs in the same color. (Clothes dryers eat socks, you know!)

Now let's take a look at the life of a blazer.

The Blazer at Work

The blazer is a hard worker in the workplace. By simply changing the colors of his shirt, tie, and slacks, a man can build almost an entire working wardrobe around a couple of blazers and a suit. One classic color is navy, but blazers can be black, brown, or any other color. Some have brass buttons, some have matching-colored buttons. Blazers come in all weights of fabrics.

If you buy a brand-name blazer from a reputable store, you should not have to worry about the quality. Watch for sales to get the best shoestring price available, and then remember to divide out the number of years you will wear the garment to determine the cost per year. Buying quality suits and blazers is an investment and makes good shoestring sense.

The Blazer at Play

Sports shirts, long or short-sleeved shirts open at the neck, or knit polo shirts with casual slacks can give the same blazer a whole new casual look. Some guys even wear a T-shirt under a blazer.

The Blazer All Dressed Up

The same blazer with a white shirt, beautiful tie, matching pocket scarf, and nice pair of tailored slacks can be worn for a dress-up evening, although a blazer will never be as formal as a suit or tuxedo.

Shoes

Most men only have one or two pairs of dress shoes at the same time: a black pair and a brown pair. They may have several pairs of casual and sports shoes. This is a very practical plan that needs no embellishment.

As we mentioned earlier, situations and workplaces vary widely. In spite of that, we will try to give you a basic plan for your workday wardrobe needs. Tweak our ideas to suit your individual needs.

For best flexibility, buy all your pants, jackets, coats, belts, shoes, and bags in your best neutral, basic colors. Then add color, whites, and prints to your wardrobe in blouses and shirts, scarves, vests, and accessories. Socks (except for dress socks) and underwear are best in white cotton. Even though white cotton socks may seem boring, they will go with all your casual clothing and will be the most comfortable socks you can wear.

PLANNING FAMILY NEEDS

Following is a list of clothing each family member might need. Consider these lists only as a place to begin planning your family's wardrobe needs. We are assuming you do laundry twice a week. If you do it more often, you may be able to get away with having fewer clothes. If you do it only once a week, you may want to increase our suggested numbers.

For Kids

The Child in Diapers—Infant to Two Years

Babies need clothing that is nonchafing, comfortable, and sturdy and gives easy access to the diaper when it needs to be changed. Pants especially need to be tough, as little ones tend to wear out the knees rather quickly. Kids may need special clothes for church and other dressy occasions. On most Sundays and in most churches, wearing clean play clothes will be fine. Kids usually play in the church nursery for a couple of hours, so let them be comfortable! For special occasions, little boys can wear a suit or slacks and dress shirt. If you can keep a tie or bow tie on him, he will look very cute. He will need dress socks and loafers or dress shoes as well. A nice cardigan or pullover sweater over a dress shirt or golf shirt paired with slacks will be acceptable for many dressy occasions.

Little girls are so fun to dress up and usually end up receiving so many cute dresses as gifts that it seems a shame not to put them in a dress when you can. Make sure the dress has no uncomfortable lace or other rough materials touching the skin. The little sweetheart will need room to move. Dresses that are too long can frustrate crawling babies and trip up walking toddlers as well. Save those for photo sessions only. Besides a cute little short dress, your little girl will need tights or underpants that are meant to cover the diaper. Many dresses come with coordinating underpants. They usually are decorated with rows of ruffles or gathered lace across the child's bottom. Choose shoes that she can walk or crawl in comfortably. The classic cute look is white or black baby doll or Mary Jane shoes. Hats, purses, and jewelry may be cute but are not appropriate for very young children. They can be a safety hazard and are too hard to keep attached. The child will usually reject them anyway. Use them with the long dress for the special photo.

For Very Young Children

5 pairs of pants or overalls
5 coordinating tops—5 long or short sleeved, depending on
    climate and season
5 undershirts
5 pairs of socks
High quality sneakers that are comfortable and give good
    support
Hat for sun protection
Light jacket
Heavy coat (in cold climates)
Snow gear—mittens, snowsuit, knit hat, boots (in cold climates)
Swimsuit

Toddlers—Preschool, Ages Two to Four

Some of you may have toddlers with their minds very set on
what they will and will not wear. Children's tastes and preferences begin to form very early in life. You may want to keep
your child with you while shopping to avoid purchasing something that the child will refuse to wear or, worse yet, will decide
to remove at the most embarrassing time. We do not suggest
overalls, as they are very frustrating for the emergency bath-
room trip. Pants should be easy for the child to undo and redo
for the same reasons. Once again, durability and comfort are the
main considerations.

For the Potty-Trained Toddler

5 pairs of pants
5 pairs of shorts, if needed in your climate
5 coordinating shirts in short or long sleeves
A warm-up suit
2 pairs of pajamas
5 pairs of underwear
5 undershirts
5 pairs of socks

1 pair of high quality sneakers
A light jacket
Heavy coat (in cold climates)
Snow gear—mittens, hat, and muffler (in cold climates)
Swimsuit
Church/dress-up clothes

School-Aged Children, Ages Five and Up

The clothing problem can become more challenging when kids reach school age. Kids discover that some labels are more prestigious than others. They see that many other kids are wearing a particular fashion and think they must have it as well. Fads and peer pressure are important to some children.

You will need to set a clothing and budget policy with your children. This may include an understanding that you will pay only so much for clothing and if they want something more expensive, they make up the difference from their own pockets.

This is the time to teach your children about Christian modesty. You may wish to ban certain clothing because of what it represents. Jo's sons do not wear T-shirts that advertise alcoholic drinks or music groups that do not share our values. Styles that relate to gangs are also debatable. Give your students biblical reasons for your guidelines. First Timothy 2:9 addresses the issue of modesty. Romans 14 speaks of how to handle debatable things and the principle of individual responsibility. Your children need parameters within which to decide what their "needs" are. Be consistent and firm, but understand their need to be like their peers and to express themselves.

If your child's school requires a uniform, it will simplify matters considerably. Uniforms are typically well made and should last long enough to be handed down to several children if properly cared for. If your school does not have some sort of system in place for trading and handing down uniforms, start the process yourself. Everyone benefits.

School dress codes vary, especially in private Christian schools. Our wardrobe guidelines assume girls may wear pants and boys may wear jeans. Denim wears better than other pants fabric choices. Your child's school clothes will last longer if they change into play clothes after school. Typically, play clothes are old school clothes that have become a bit ratty, worn, stained, or otherwise inappropriate for school.

For School-Aged Boys

2–3 pairs of jeans in good repair
5–7 tops for winter, 5–7 tops for summer
Underwear
Something to sleep in
Swimsuit
2–3 pairs of shorts
Old shirts for play
Old jeans for play
Light jacket
Warm-up suit
Cold weather coat, gloves, hat, muffler, boots (in cold climates)
6 pairs of athletic socks
Good quality sneakers
Belt (optional)
Special sports wear
Church/special occasion attire: suit, blazer and slacks, or sweater and slacks; tie (may be able to use one of Dad's); dress shirt; belt or suspenders; dress socks (may be able to use Dad's); dress shoes

For School-Aged Girls

5 pairs of pants: jeans, slacks, or overalls
5–7 tops for winter, 5–7 tops for summer

Underwear
7 pairs of socks
Sneakers
Belts (optional)
Light jacket
Cold weather coat, hat, gloves, muffler (in cold climates)
Swimsuit
4–5 pairs of shorts
Old pants for play
Old shirts for play
Warm-up suit
Something to sleep in
Special sports attire
Church/special occasion attire: pretty dress or skirt and
   blouse; slip; tights or pretty socks; dress shoes; coordinat-
   ing hair bow or ribbon; handbag (optional)

For the Woman

A woman's basic wardrobe depends greatly on where she works and how many special occasions she must dress up for. A simple, classic dress (black or brown, depending on what looks good on you) with pearls and matching pumps will work for many occasions. Paired with different jackets, vests, jewelry, and shoes, it can go to the opera, the company Christmas party, or a dinner party.

For the Office

2 suits in neutral colors
1 jacket in becoming color
3 skirts that coordinate with the jacket or with one of the suit
   jackets
1 pair of trousers in neutral color
Dress that can be paired with one of the jackets
5 blouses that coordinate with suits and jackets

Cardigan sweater in a neutral color
Belts
Scarves
A light neutral-colored pair of pumps
A dark neutral-colored pair of pumps
Hose in skin tones
Overcoat

Most of these clothes could also be considered "business casual," although she may need more pairs of dress trousers and fewer skirts and might want a couple of pairs of flat shoes to wear with pants. Business casual for women may include jumpers with turtle necks or simple jackets with zippers.

For Informal Workplace and Off-Hours

Jeans
Twill or canvas slacks
Shorts
T-shirts
Camp style or golf shirts
Turtleneck shirts
Warm-up suit
Swimsuit
Something to sleep in
Robe
Athletic socks
Trouser socks
Light jacket
Cold weather coat, gloves, hat, muffler (in cold climates)
Belt

For the Man

A man's basic wardrobe is also determined by where he works, his company's policy on business casual or more formal business attire, and how many special occasions he must dress up for. For most special occasions a suit that might be worn to the office or church will do the job. If you need a tuxedo often, buy one. Some professions require frequent use of a black or nearly black suit.

For the Office

Gray flannel suit
Navy blue suit
Tweed or small-checked jacket (to wear with suit pants or camel pants)
Camel wool slacks (wear with blue suit jacket or separate jacket)
Seven dress shirts in solid colors and pinstripes
Ties
Dress socks
Shoes—brogues, oxfords, or nice loafers
Belt
Suspenders

For a business casual workplace, a man can wear plaid or conservatively patterned shirts (not tropical prints), turtlenecks, and sweaters. In some workplaces where business casual is the policy, a man's shirts must have a collar, but he does not need to wear a tie. Pants can be dress pants, nice khakis, or cotton slacks but not jeans. Jeans and T-shirts are reserved for a completely casual day such as "casual Friday."

For the Informal Workplace and Off-Hours

Jeans
Khaki tan slacks
Denim shorts
Khaki walking shorts
T-shirts
Golf shirts
Long-sleeved shirts in plain colors, plaid, or prints

Blue chambray work shirts
Belt
Athletic socks
Sneakers
Safety shoes (if required in workplace)
Casual leather shoes—moccasins, loafers
Swimsuit
Warm-up suit
Sleepwear
Robe

We've said it before and we'll say it again: We believe it pays to buy quality clothing. The next chapter will teach you more on that subject. You may have fewer clothes, but if they fit right, are in a becoming style and color, and are of good quality, they will save you a lot of money, and you will know you look great!

Shoestring Tips

1. Get each family member's colors analyzed.
2. Carry a small notebook with everyone's needs and sizes listed.
3. Get rid of things that are not your colors or are not becoming.
4. Try on clothing in front of a full-length mirror and in good light to fully analyze whether or not it is becoming.
5. Look in a full-length mirror to determine if you need to bulk up a body part or need to practice diminishing tactics.
6. If you have large hips, remove side pockets from skirts and slacks and carefully sew the openings shut.
7. Begin to collect basic clothing in your best neutral colors.
8. Sell those nice things that are not becoming to you at a consignment shop.

9. Add shoulder pads to tops if your hips are wider than your chest. Remove shoulder pads if you have broad shoulders or narrow hips.

10. Make your husband clean out his wallet and carry less in those bulgy pockets.

11. If part of a suit or outfit doesn't fit right or is unbecoming, mix and match it with something else.

12. Use a vest over a simple shirt to add bulk to a top or hide the fact that your waist is a bit large.

13. Trade clothing with someone your size who has made shopping mistakes similar to yours. For example, if you are a winter, give that beige suit to a spring—maybe she has a navy blue blouse she never wears.

14. Add extras to what you have. Sometimes the difference between an ordinary garment and a designer garment is little more than the embellishments that have been added to the designer garment. You can add these little touches to personalize a garment and make it look as though you bought it from the most expensive boutique shop in town. Trims, appliqués, sequins, beading, and decorative stitches all bring value to a garment but are not hard to add.

FOUR

SHOES, PURSES, AND ACCESSORIES

If you are old enough, you may remember Imelda Marcos—the wife of Philippine president Ferdinand Marcos. When he was indicted for embezzlement and asked to leave his home in the 1980s, the media discovered that Imelda, a well-known clotheshorse, had spent some of that embezzled money purchasing a closetful of shoes—over a thousand pairs, actually. She was the laughingstock of the world when the story broke.

However, some of us seem to have a similar mind-set. Something in our psyche must be fixed by having a lot of shoes! We collect shoes in every style and every color. We never get rid of any. Every outfit requires a matching pair of shoes. Some people spend hundreds of dollars on every pair in their huge collection, while the average shoe-aholic may spend only a few dollars whenever she sees a two-for-one sale. Deep down, we understand Imelda Marcos. We just use our own cash instead of someone else's.

Our experience tells us that a lot of people have too many pairs of shoes crowding their closets, even if they are not shoe-aholics. You may own many pairs of shoes but often lack the appropriate or perfect pair for every occasion. In addition, belts, scarves, and other miscellaneous accessories may be cluttering up your closet. Your jewelry box may be a jumbled mess of things you never wear. It is time to go through all this stuff and get it organized and get rid of what doesn't belong in your newly organized, coordinated wardrobe. Analyze each item. Does it fit your style and lifestyle?

The accessories we wear add individuality to our wardrobe. By adding a different piece of jewelry and a belt to an outfit, we can give that outfit a whole new look. While some accessories may be categorized as frivolous, some are truly necessary. For example, most scarves serve merely to add a dash of color and style to an outfit. But when a wool jacket rubs your neck uncomfortably, a scarf becomes a necessity. Belts can draw the eye to a person's trim waist, but many men truly need a belt to hold up their pants.

In this chapter we will talk about choosing and shopping for belts, shoes, purses, ties, briefcases, jewelry, and other accessories. We will help you figure out what your minimal needs are and how to spot quality. You will find that this chapter complements and completes our wardrobe guidelines from chapters 2 and 3. Once again, you must consider your specific lifestyle, personal style, and coloring as well as any special needs.

Once you have organized the wardrobe of family members to reflect who they are, what their needs are, and what is most becoming to them, you will discover that not only are fewer clothing items needed but fewer accessories as well. For example, a Romantic-style girl with spring coloring will not need day-glow orange sneakers because she will have nothing to match them. You will discover that you really only need a few pairs of shoes in basic colors that work with your wardrobe. Your closets and dresser drawers will be emptier but, surprisingly, you will have more to wear.

Rather than just telling you how to choose and shop for accessories, we will follow five fictitious friends who know how to choose the right accessories while shopping at their favorite shoestring locations. These individuals are savvy shoppers and know a good deal when they see one. Each one represents one of our five styles, and they also span our four color categories.

Let us begin with Chip, a twenty-year-old man who epitomizes the Sporty-Casual style and whose coloring fits neatly into the summer category. With him is his girlfriend, Linda, a slim, winter Classic.

CHIP AND LINDA
ON A SHOPPING DATE

Chip doesn't go shopping very often but he has set aside today to acquire a few necessities. He is going to conquer! On his list are hiking boots, something to keep his head warm on winter jaunts, and a warm vest. He also enjoys spending as much time as possible with Linda, who hopes to find a few accessories that will help her make the transition from college student to first grade teacher in a few months. She is already collecting a basic working wardrobe.

Chip has mapped out their day to hit a few promising yard sales, a couple of thrift stores, and his favorite discount sporting goods store. They carry cash not only to make shopping quicker and easier but also to limit their spending. When their cash is gone, they are done.

The first few yard sales were dead ends for Chip. He found a few pairs of cheap, imitation leather hiking boots and a quilted vest with snaps missing, but he passed all those up. Imitation leather is not good for his feet because it doesn't breathe. He has no idea how to replace snaps and doesn't want to learn. But while Chip found nothing he wanted, Linda found a pair of gold-tone button earrings that looked like new. She will disinfect them before wearing them. Since they are young (and in love), visiting five yard sales with such meager results doesn't discourage them.

At the sixth yard sale Chip spots a red, quilted down vest hiding in a rack full of prom gowns. He tries it on. It fits like it was made for him. He even likes the color. He notices that a company known for quality outdoor clothing manufactured it. The price? Ten dollars. Although Chip had planned to spend more than ten dollars for a vest, he cannot resist haggling. The sellers and Chip settle on $7.50.

Across the street at another yard sale, Linda comes across a gold mine. Someone who used to be her size and who shares her style and coloring is getting rid of beautiful genuine leather belts! Linda's trim waist is one of her best features, so as she shops she keeps an eye open for interesting belts. Obviously this seller not only has good taste but also shares Linda's contempt for accessories made of plastic or vinyl. Linda tries on several belts and inspects them for problems before buying them, of course. One of the belts is just a bit snug, and she knows that would never be comfortable or look good, so she rejects it. She picks up a shiny, narrow black belt, a similar red belt, and a wide, flashy, sequined belt—all for five dollars.

She is sure she will wear the black and red belts often but is not sure if she will have a lot of opportunities to use the sequined belt, especially as long as she is dating Chip, the outdoorsman. In her mind's eye she can see how this flashy belt would transform her black wool pants and black silk blouse into evening clothing. She hopes to find a basic black dress soon, and the belt could dress that up as well. She decides to buy it anyway since the belt is so cheap and dressy occasions do come up. In the back of her mind, Linda acknowledges that her roommate may have many occasions to borrow it.

As they visit several more yard sales, Linda picks up a beautiful navy-and-white striped silk scarf for $2.50. Chip rejects some worn hiking boots. If the boots had been nearly new, he might have been interested, but they had been worn enough to conform to the previous wearer's feet. They would never feel comfortable on anyone else's feet. He does, however, find a beautiful silk tie that looks as though it has never been worn.

At the first thrift store, Goodwill, Chip checks out the men's hats but finds nothing. He looks in the women's department because sometimes things are not put where they belong. Lo and behold, there he finds the perfect hat. It is a blue knit made of wool but lined with cotton. Chip gingerly tries it on, not knowing who wore it last or how clean the last wearer was. The fit is comfortable and the tags say it is hand washable. He will wash it as soon as he gets home. He checks out the shoe department. Still no hiking boots.

Linda rejects the scarves she finds here. There was a nice silk scarf, but it wasn't her colors. She does find a classically designed black leather purse in amazingly good shape. She thoroughly inspects her potential purchase, trying all the zippers, investigating every pocket. She found a ten-dollar bill in a purse pocket at a thrift store once, so she always checks. There is a small tear in the lining that she is sure she can easily mend by hand. (*Thank you, Mom, for teaching me how to sew!*) She also picks up a simple satin evening bag that looks new. With proper care and not too much use, this little bag will get her through many dressy special occasions.

At the next thrift store, Linda finds some good wooden shoe trees. She knows that her new work shoes will last longer and look good longer if she keeps them polished, does not wear the same pair every day, and keeps shoe trees in them. Chip still has not found a pair of hiking boots.

Our smart young shoppers stop at a nearby park to eat the picnic lunch Linda packed (she has found the sure path to Chip's heart!). Since they have been fast and focused, they have covered a lot of ground in one morning. They get ready to make their way to one more thrift store and then the sporting goods store.

At the Salvation Army thrift store, they find an unadvertised sale in progress. All clothing and accessories are ninety-nine cents. They carefully check out the footwear. Still no good hiking boots. However, Linda finds a brand-new pair of black leather pumps in her size. She passes up the royal blue ones, the pink and green ones, and the tan ones. She will not clutter her closet with things that do not fit her style and coloring, and at this point in her wardrobe-building, she needs things in neutral colors first. She knows that she will need two pairs of low-heeled leather shoes for her future career. Wearing the same pair every day is hard on one's feet and hard on the shoes. Maybe after she has a complete basic wardrobe she will be able to afford some extra things. Chip finds a pair of nice ski gloves that he cannot live without for ninety-nine cents. Okay, so they were not on his list, but they should have been. And who could pass up such a deal?

Finally they make their weary way to the sporting goods discount store ten miles south of the city. Chip just wants to get there and find some hiking boots. One of the reasons Chip chose this day to shop was because of the clearance sale at this store. Their already great prices are discounted even more.

Chip is not disappointed. The hiking boots of his dreams are on clearance. It takes some hunting in the messy stacks of boots to find matching left and right boots in his size, but he does. For a mere twenty dollars his shoe wardrobe is now complete. At home the new boots will sit neatly beside his brown leather loafers (kept in shape with shoe trees, of course) and his sneakers on a shoe rack in his closet.

Linda finds, for only $3.99, a black felt hat to wear on winter outings with Chip. And so our young couple completes their shopping with cash left over for pizza. Maybe they will even live happily ever after!

A MOTHER AND DAUGHTER OUTING

Our next shopping expedition is with Cleo and her daughter Amelia. These two are as different as a mother and daughter can be. Cleo, a tall but no longer extremely thin "winter," looks stunning when she wears her favorite High Fashion–Dramatic fashions. Sweet, petite, ten-year-old Amelia loves to dress in Romantic clothing in hues that best set off her blond hair and spring coloring. In spite of their fashion differences, these two have found a common ground in shopping for accessories. They not only enjoy finding things they like for themselves, but they also derive great satisfaction in discovering items the other will like.

Like our previous pair, Cleo and Amelia begin their shopping at yard sales and then thrift stores. They plan to end up at the Nordstrom's Rack store. Cleo packed a lunch while Amelia filled two water bottles. They hope to find a good deal on black pumps for Cleo, some accessories to spice up her wardrobe, and some hair doodads and shoes for Amelia. They are open to other serendipitous finds as long as their cash holds out after buying what they need.

At the first yard sale, Amelia's eye is drawn to a table covered with costume jewelry. Among the plastic junk, the small stud earrings, and the cute little necklaces, she finds some wonderful costume jewelry that is bold and beautiful. Not everyone can wear this stuff, but she knows that her mom can wear it with dash and style. While none of it is solid gold, the gold finish is still in good shape on a couple of large pins and a pair of earrings. What really catches Cleo's trained eye, though, is a pair of large sterling silver earrings badly in need of polishing. The tarnished finish hides a real treasure. Does the seller realize what

81

she is offering for only a dollar? Cleo walks away with a lot of jewelry for only six dollars.

A couple of yard sales later, Cleo discovers a bunch of hair accessories that will look so pretty in her daughter's long blond hair. The person having the yard sale makes hair bows and headbands for a small shop in town. She is offering them at a steep discount at her yard sale. Cleo helps her daughter choose a few things that will look good and match what she already owns. They buy a Christmas bow to be worn later in the year.

Many yard sales offer kids' shoes for sale, but Cleo is very picky about what her children wear for running and playing. Her pediatrician told her that kids need arch support, plenty of toe room, and ankle support when they are very young. The wider the sole on the shoe, the easier her toddlers can stay on their feet. Cleo sees plenty of the cheap sneakers that have cartoon and movie characters, but she turns up her nose at these. They may be cute, but they are not quality or good for Amelia's feet. However, Cleo does find some rubber flip-flop sandals for the beach that look hardly worn. Her kids do not spend a lot of time in flip-flops, but a pair does come in handy.

At other yard sales they pick up a broad-brimmed black felt hat for Cleo, some new (still in the package) ivory lace tights for Amelia, and a lovely silk scarf in splashes of claret, black, and white for Cleo. At one sale they find some cute snow boots for Amelia and her older brother. Winter seems far away but it is smart to think ahead, you know. Cleo will store the boots in a "winter" box until they are needed. She also finds a black umbrella for her husband that just needs a little repair. She knows she can do the repair.

Feeling recharged after eating their sack lunches, they go on to the thrift stores, hoping to find some shoes. So far Cleo hasn't found any new or even almost-new black pumps in her size or any shoes for Amelia. Her luck is no better at the thrift stores today. But while searching through all the imitation leather belts, she does find a wide, maroon, genuine leather belt that is just one inch too big. The buckle and belt are in good shape. Since it only costs three dollars and she will pay just a dollar more to have a couple more holes punched in it at her neighborhood shoe repair shop, Cleo buys it. A nice, properly fitting belt sets off an outfit so beautifully. They also purchase a woven, brown canvas belt that Amelia needs for school.

Finally, at Nordstrom's Rack they spend quite a bit of time searching through the many pairs of shoes displayed. Cleo will not buy just any pair of shoes. She has a mental checklist of qualities that every pair of shoes in her closet must meet. They must fit well, be comfortable, be her style, be in good repair, be in fashion, be made of leather or other natural materials, coordinate with her wardrobe, and not be like other shoes she already owns. This keeps down the clutter in her closet and makes it easier to put together an outfit.

The mother and daughter study every pair of black shoes in Cleo's size. They also check the sizes just above and below hers because some manufacturers cut their shoes a bit big or a bit small. Today they are fortunate to find a lovely pair of low-heeled black leather pumps in the size she usually wears that fit beautifully. They cost only a fraction of their original retail price.

Since they are here, they check out the shoes in girls' sizes. Cleo's demands for her daughter's footwear are the same as hers, plus she wants plenty of space for Amelia's toes to wiggle, a bit of growing room, and good arch support. They bypass the sneakers made of vinyl, even if they are very cute. They find a pair of name-brand sneakers that meet all their criteria. Amelia runs around the store a bit to see if the shoes are comfortable. She tells her mom that they are very comfy and she also thinks they help her run faster. Cleo notices that the shoes do not slip at the heel. She decides to purchase them. They cost more than the vinyl ones but they will last longer, be much more comfortable, and be much better for Amelia's growing feet.

The plain white sneakers do not excite Amelia but some black patent leather shoes with bows on the toes do. They do not fulfill all the criteria for good shoes because they are made of vinyl and have no arch support. But since they will only be worn for an hour or two a week at the most and are very inexpensive and Amelia does need some dress shoes, Cleo buys them.

Cleo also checks out the bag, purse, and briefcase department. She is looking for something that looks businesslike, will hold her personal items, and can double as a briefcase. She is not sure what she wants, so she is still in the shopping stage to see what is available and what will work for her when she begins her new part-time job next week.

Mother and daughter return home pleased with their purchases and full of fond memories of their day together. Three months later we join Cleo's cousin Autumn, who is shopping with two old friends she is visiting with near Colorado Springs, Stu and Lisa. Let's see what they come up with on their shopping expedition.

An Autumn Outing

Several decades ago when Autumn was born, her parents were inspired by her time of birth and the color of her baby hair to name her as they did. The name has been a perfect fit. Auburn-haired Autumn wears fall colors beautifully in her Artsy-Creative style. While wandering through the wonderful shops along Old Colorado City's main street with her friends, she keeps her eyes open for the kind of jewelry and scarves she enjoys wearing.

As the three old friends walk past a window, they all gasp in unison at the sight of some truly unique hand-painted scarves artfully draped on mannequins. Inside the shop they find the artist herself. The shop carries not only scarves but shawls and vests as well. And many of them seem to be in Autumn's colors. The three friends look through the selections and find a tan scarf and brown vest that are painted with copper and gold designs. Stu and Lisa buy the vest and the scarf. Autumn suddenly knows what she is getting for her birthday tomorrow!

In a junky antique store that was too quirky to resist, they unearth more treasures. Autumn digs through a big basket of clearance items and comes up with a long string of large Russian amber beads with matching earrings. Her daughter, who shares her coloring and style, will love these for Christmas. Knowing that Autumn's husband often uses a cane to walk, Stu points out a box full of interesting walking sticks and canes. The man has style! Autumn chooses a hand-carved beauty that will be a great Christmas present.

As they are leaving the antique shop, Autumn's large macramé bag catches on a sign and dumps everything helter-skelter all over the sidewalk. Lipstick tubes and coins roll into the gutter. Tissues blow away in the wind. Pencils, pens, paperclips, notes written on restaurant napkins, cosmetics, her checkbook, credit cards, and much more tell passersby that an unorganized person is having trouble. Autumn is more than a little embarrassed at the mess and the amount of stuff she carries.

After everything is picked up and stashed back in the copious bag, the three friends find a bench. Lisa dumps the contents of her purse next to her on the bench. Not much falls out. As she puts it back she explains to her friend how she keeps her purse organized. There is a place for everything and everything is in its place. A wallet holds all her cash, checkbook, cards, and pictures of the grandkids, a small notepad, and a pen. A small, zippered bag holds her cosmetics and facial tissues. There is a pocket for her reading glasses and another one for her keys. Lisa admits that she cleans out her purse twice a month when she pays bills. Autumn is impressed and vows that she will find a purse, wallet, and cosmetic purse like that. She has had one too many embarrassing moments when her purse has overturned. She smells something good from a nearby café and suggests lunch.

After lunch they resume their shopping. They pass several shops that sell jewelry but only one that really catches the eyes of the three friends. The jewelry in this shop is fashioned from bits of rocks and shells artfully entwined with copper wire. Each piece is a unique work of art. Autumn, an artist herself, appreciates the craftsmanship. She uses the cash she set aside for just such a find to purchase the latest addition to her jewelry collection. She dons the jewelry immediately as it goes so well with what she is wearing. She looks and feels fabulous.

Autumn sees one more store she wants to visit. Stu says he will wait on a handy bench while the two ladies finish their shopping. The smell of leather emanates from the Killed a Kow shop. Lisa has a pretty good idea what Autumn is looking for here. Yep. She heads straight for the purses. The two friends inspect every brown purse to see what it offers. They decide on a nice reddish brown one that is a little bigger than Lisa's but has just as many compartments and just happens to be on sale. The wallet selection is a little easier and cheaper. Autumn buys both the purse and matching wallet, then asks where she might find a cosmetic bag. Two stores down the street they purchase a small, plastic, zippered bag for $1.79. Then Autumn and Lisa join Stu on the bench and change everything from Autumn's macramé bag to the new purse, wallet, and bag. A lot of things end up in the trash. Autumn feels so organized.

The three friends are not as young as they used to be, so they are done for the day. Each feels good about his or her purchases. After years of learning from their mistakes, they are much smarter shoppers than they were as young adults, so they should not feel any "buyer's regret" tonight. We hope they shared all that wisdom with their children!

The Continuing Saga of Sally and Her Wardrobe

After cleaning out her closet, our poor friend Sally Frazzle is left with only one simple tan dress, Old Faithful. Unfortunately, Sally's schedule requires her to dress up and be with the same people for five days in a row. Smart Sally can use her collection of accessories and a few pieces from her limited but coordinated wardrobe to transform Old Faithful into a different outfit every day. Let's see how she pulls off this miracle.

Day One

On day one Sally is not feeling her usual Romantic self. The day's schedule looks very businesslike. Sally pairs the dress with a brown blazer, brown pumps, and a brown belt with a simple gold-toned buckle. Her only jewelry is a pair of gold knot earrings and a thin gold chain with a cross pendant. She looks so together!

Day Two

For day two, Sally wears a cream turtleneck under the dress and follows the cream theme through with her belt and shoes. Her jewelry is the only thing that shows that at heart she is truly a Romantic. She wears a golden necklace with a cameo pendant and matching earrings. So very pretty today!

Day Three

Sally gets a little more daring for day three. She is feeling very High Fashion–Dramatic today. A leopard print silk scarf she found at a yard sale inspired the feeling. She wears it around her neck with a full, puffy knot in front and the ends hanging down the front of her dress. Her brown belt and shoes are used again but she gets a little bolder with her jewelry. Large earrings made of ivory and wood and a coordinating bracelet bring out the jungle theme of her outfit. Striking!

That evening Sally finds a one-hour dry cleaner so her dress is fresh for day four.

Day Four

Another garage sale scarf inspires Sally's Artsy-Creative look for day four. This long, thin scarf is in a bold print of cream, brown, rust, and tan. Sally ties it around her waist as a belt. She sets off the whole outfit with a costume jewelry set of earrings, necklace, and bracelet that is big and clunky, made of wooden beads dyed to similar tones as the scarf interspersed with gold and bronze beads. Sally found the beads and jewelry makings on sale at a craft store. Her cream pumps seem to work perfectly with this outfit. And again, Sally looks so attractive!

Day Five

Day five finds Sally getting a little tired of this dress but still doing her creative wardrobe magic. Today she puts a brown suede vest over the dress. She bought a brown western-style belt at a thrift store to give the outfit a western flair. Silver-and-turquoise southwestern-style jewelry that she found at a bargain price on their New Mexico vacation last summer are the perfect finishing touch. Her brown pumps coordinate with the brown vest and belt. She looks ready to face any trouble the wild world can throw her way.

Every day Sally has looked fashionable and well put together. She actually simply copied what she saw while window shopping at high quality department stores and boutiques. That is also how she found the dress and shoes that she wears with such confidence and flair.

SHOESTRING TIPS

1. Use dickeys under sweaters, dresses, and jackets. A dickey is basically a decorative collar without a shirt. You can make dickeys from patterns available from all the major pattern companies, buy them from department stores, or check out the shoestring sources. You can also buy a blouse at a shoestring source, or take one of your own blouses, and cut away everything but the part that will form the dickey.

2. Dress up a basic long-sleeved dress by making lace bracelet cuffs.

3. Use scarves to add a lot of impact, style, and color to a woman's outfit.

4. Watch for leather belts at shoestring places. When people put on inches and give up their belts, you benefit.

5. Buy buckles and belt-making supplies at a fabric store and make your own belts. They carry kits for making fabric belts, belt webbing in many colors, and all kinds of belt buckles.

6. Make a lovely belt by buying a few inches of ultrasuede fabric. Just purchase two or three inches of fabric in the width of the bolt and knot it around your waist or tie the two ends in a bow. Ultrasuede needs no finishing as it will not ravel.

7. Use a fabric rectangle as a sari, headdress, sarong, or shawl.

8. Buy a few good classic pieces of jewelry and a gold watch and wear them with everything.

9. Avoid trendy accessories.

FIVE

SHOPPING FOR QUALITY

This business of clothing your family on a shoestring budget is not about cheap. It's not about buying shoes, jeans, and under- and outerwear because they are on sale. It is not about looking as if you walked out of a closeout basement where you grabbed items with no thought about style or quality. No, this book is about buying clothing that is quality, has classic staying power, is well constructed so that it survives both the washing machine and the hard wear, and gives the one wearing the clothing a sense of style. Clothing purchased on a shoestring budget doesn't mean your family looks as if they were caught in an explosion at a thrift shop.

Over the years Jo has learned the benefit of buying quality. She only has two pairs of dress shoes in her closet, and she has owned them for fifteen years. She does not need to use them very often in her lifestyle, but when she does she can always wear them with confidence. These fine leather low-heeled shoes cost her a bundle, even on sale, because they are of great quality. They have been worth every penny. She has taken good care of them and therefore they have lasted a long time.

Jo also bought some black wool dress trousers about the same time she bought her long-lasting dress shoes. These very nice lined pants still fit quite nicely, thank you. Jo gets them out of storage every winter for dressier occasions. Buying quality has paid off.

We are told that bank tellers are taught to recognize counterfeit money not by looking at counterfeit money but by handling real money. We learn to spot excellent quality and style by studying excellent quality and style. So even though this book is about learning how to dress well on a tight budget, we're going to recommend that you visit stores where top quality merchandise is sold. While you are learning what makes a quality garment, you will also learn which brand names always provide the best quality. Then you will recognize those brands in your shoestring wanderings.

Looking for Quality

Once you've found a garment you like and that fits you and your lifestyle, you don't want it falling apart the first time you wash it. Enter quality. You've heard it said that you get what you pay for, and that is often true if you are shopping the regular retail stores. But when you are thrift, consignment, or outlet shopping for clothing, you want quality without spending a lot of money.

Quality means the best of design, fabric, and workmanship. With the amount of clothing being manufactured today, much of it of low quality, it seems as if the idea is to throw clothing away as soon as it needs cleaning. But that's not what you want to do if saving money is a priority. You want longevity and a garment that will still have style and still be in one piece years later. Let's run down the checklist of what makes for quality so that when you find that perfect royal blue suit at your favorite shoestring place, you have something against which to measure its quality.

Seams

When you find a garment you like and that seems to fit all your criteria, start inspecting it by looking at the seams. Are they straight? Are the stitches close together? Have the stitches come out and the seams popped open anyplace? If a seam is popped open, can you easily mend it or take it someplace to be mended? The shoulder seam of a coat or jacket is tough to get to in order to mend a rip, so it's probably not worth your time to fix it. Keep looking.

Turn the garment inside out. How are the seams finished? Have the edges begun to unravel? Could you take care of that problem? Is there a large enough seam allowance so that if the garment needs letting out you can do it? Does the fabric have a hard finish that will show the old seam line if you let it out?

Hems

Does the hem appear flat and smooth from the outside? Is the garment the right length or does it need to be altered? You can always shorten a garment, but will the fabric of this garment allow you to let it down? In most cases you cannot let down hems without a crease showing. Gwen once heard a funny story about a mother who let down the hems on her daughter's dresses. She did it so often that when the girl got a dress that hadn't been let down, the mother got a pencil and drew a line on the skirt to simulate a let-down hem.

We've seen some pretty innovative and totally ineffective ways of shortening a skirt. Some people just turn the hem up and stitch it in place. That makes about three thicknesses of fabric.

It looks bulky. It looks puckered. It looks *awful!* Some folks have taken the hem out first and then turned up the whole thing without cutting down the width of the hem. That four-inch hem looks awful too. Others have cut the hem off and turned it back, but the method they have used to take care of the raw edge (usually stretch lace) looks terrible too. Or they didn't use anything over the raw edge of the hem at all, so there it is, loose threads and all. When we get to the remodeling and sewing chapter, we'll talk about some options for hems and how to do it right, but begin by inspecting your clothing find for bad hems.

Collars and Cuffs

Check the condition of the collar and cuffs, especially on used garments. Are they frayed? Are they soiled beyond what can be cleaned by washing? Could you take the collar off and leave just the band? Could you replace the cuffs or cut them off and add trim in their place? Could you cut off the sleeves and make it a short-sleeved garment? Is the garment worth the trouble?

Collars on a quality garment will lie flat without buckling or gapping at the throat. The left side will be the same length and size as the right. On poorly made garments, the underside of the collar is often larger than the top, so it bunches up. Sometimes the stiffening material inside the collar comes loose and causes rippling on the top of the collar. Don't buy such a garment. There is no way to reattach that inner material to the collar fabric. On a quality garment, trim will be sewn on with care and precision. Sometimes the collar underneath the trim is well made and in good condition, but the trim either is worn or was never of good quality in the first place. Could you remove the trim? Or replace the trim? Be sure to try on the garment. An uncomfortable collar is a miserable thing to have around your neck.

Perhaps the garment is a dress with a scoop neck. Try on the dress to ensure it doesn't scoop farther than you want it to. While facing a mirror, bend over. Look up and into the mirror while you are bent over. Does the garment pass the modesty test? Also check to see that the facing is firmly attached and won't roll to the outside.

Sleeves

Have the sleeves been set in carefully with no puckers? Check the elbows. Are they worn? Would a leather elbow patch add style to the jacket and fix the problem at the same time? If the garment has lining, does it fit well? The lining should not hang down lower than the hem of the sleeve or be much bigger or smaller than the garment. Is it worn? Can it be replaced? Would you want to do that?

Gwen once purchased a new linen suit at a thrift shop. There was something wrong with the lining in the sleeve. Since it was only one sleeve, she was sure it wouldn't be hard to fix even if she had to replace the whole sleeve lining. When she took out the stitching at the cuff, she discovered that the lining had been twisted a couple of times before being sewn in place. All she had to do was remove some stitches, untwist the lining, and reattach it at the cuff. Voila! A gorgeous linen suit for a song—well, for a stitch.

Waistbands

Check the waistband. Does it twist, fold over, or roll up? How will you be wearing the garment? If it will be worn with a belt, the waistband won't matter so much, but if the waist—your waist—is to be on display, the waistband needs to be smooth and fit you well. If everything fits but the waistband and you really like the garment, could you alter the waistband? Is there enough fabric to let it out? If you need to take it in, you will not have such a big problem unless it is more than an inch or so.

Because you are not spending a lot on the garment, you can afford to take it to a professional tailor for altering if you cannot do it yourself. Even if you hire someone to alter the garment, you will still save a bundle.

Zippers and Plackets

Check to see how the zipper looks. Does it lay flat or is the fabric puckered over the zipper either because it was improperly sewn in or because the fabric has shrunk or stretched? Slide the pull up and down. Does it work smoothly or hang up? Will the zipper slowly unzip itself while being worn? Zippers can be replaced easily either by yourself or by a seamstress. Jo recently had a zipper replaced in a pair of Al's trousers by a seamstress for only seven dollars. See if the placket is properly stitched down. This, too, is an easy fix. If the zipper is the hidden kind, is it truly hidden or bulging out of its hiding place?

Buttonholes

Bound buttonholes used to be a sure mark of quality in a garment. They have not been used much in the last few years, but it is our understanding that they are making a comeback. Until they do come back, check machine-worked buttonholes on garments carefully. Are the threads frayed or beginning to fray? Have puckers or gaps been created with sloppy sewing in the buttonholes? Is this something you can fix? Do you want to take the time to do so?

Buttons

Buttons are the jewelry of clothing and, as such, can be changed on a whim. There are gorgeous buttons available. Some of them are expensive, but if you find a great deal on a quality garment and either hate the buttons or just want to change them, then even with the most expensive buttons the total price of the garment is still low.

Gwen has a navy blue double-breasted blazer she made and has worn for years. It had plain navy buttons for a long time. Then she visited a lighthouse in California where the gift shop was selling replicas of lighthouse keepers' buttons. She bought some and replaced her plain buttons. A little gold braid on the sleeves, a crest on the pocket, and she has gotten another nine years out of the garment. She gets more compliments on that jacket than almost anything she owns.

Another time Gwen bought a new dress at a thrift shop. It had twelve big gold-rimmed pearl buttons all the way down the front. Two of them were missing, which explained why the dress was at the thrift shop. Gwen knew that replacing all those buttons would be very expensive. So to solve the problem, first she moved the bottom two buttons to the top because the top buttons were the most visible. Then she went to a fabric store and searched and searched for buttons of similar size and style. But alas, she could not find quite the right thing. So it was time for a little inventiveness. First she found some pearl buttons that were about the same size as the center of the buttons on the dress. Then she located some flat gold buttons that were just a little larger than the pearl buttons. The pearl buttons had a shank. She drilled a hole in the gold button, put the shank of the pearl button through it, and sewed the whole "button" to the dress. Because those two buttons were at the bottom of the dress and because people aren't very observant, it worked. Gwen got a new dress for very little and replacement buttons for a couple of dollars.

Soil, Stains, Pulls in Fabric

Check carefully, particularly on used garments, for soiling or stains. Some of these will come out in the washing machine or can be removed by the dry cleaner, but many will not. If you "know your stains" and are sure you can get them out and the price is right—cheap—go ahead and buy the garment. Some stains may be hidden with patches or pockets—we'll tell you more about that trick in chapter 8.

Gwen has a beautiful turquoise silk caftan with gold threads. When she spotted it in a thrift shop, she saw that it was badly stained. Since it was only five dollars, she decided to buy it. At home, she washed it in the washing machine using the gentle cycle and soap made especially for silk. Every trace of the stain came out. The heavy gold embroidery shrank up some in the washing machine, but she was able to stretch and press it. The result is a beautiful garment she wears as a hostess gown. She was pretty sure the stain would come out, but if it had not, she had not spent much on the garment.

Don't buy a garment with perspiration stains. They probably will never come out. Wine and coffee stains are tricky, so you might want to consult a stain removal guide. Lipstick can be removed, as can other grease-based stains. You will find a lot more help in library books than we can provide in our limited space.

As an industrial worker, Gwen's father got his work clothing very greasy. Her mother would work vegetable shortening into the grease stain and rub it hard. The shortening would loosen the petroleum-based stain. Then she would work in detergent, and the stain would come out in the wash. You probably would not want to try this method on clothing with man-made fibers in it, but it works great on cotton denim and chambray.

A surefire way to know the age of a used garment is to look at the little tag that gives fabric content and size. If it is crisp and readable, the garment has not been washed much. If it is tattered and unreadable, the garment is older. If it is a quality garment that you like, the age probably does not matter much. Just take a good look at the style of an older garment. If it is a classic, it is probably still in style. If it is a trendy garment and has been washed a lot, it probably looks as if it has been dragged behind a car. You do not want it.

Inspecting Knits for Quality

In the case of sweaters and other knits, your quality inspection needs to be slightly different. First of all, check the fiber content of the knitted garment. Wool holds it shape and will last much longer than man-made fibers. Man-made fibers tend to "pill" more than wool, and even if a wool fabric does pill, those pills can be removed effectively with sweater stones or other tools made for that purpose. (More about fibers later in this chapter.) Hold the garment up to see if it sags or bags. If it does not hang well now, it never will. Is it lined? Lining stabilizes the garment and is a mark of quality.

Cotton knits are cool and comfortable, and we all live in them, but they fade and get old looking rather quickly. That goes for sweaters as well as T-shirts. If a worn look doesn't bother you, you will find thousands of shirts out there to be had for a few pennies. A faded cotton sweater can be dyed to revive its vivid color.

When it comes to cotton T-shirts, you may find it best to buy them new. They are not terribly expensive if you purchase them from discount stores. Some of the mass marketers have seasonal sales of T-shirts. They are well made, durable, and comfortable. Gwen's daughter buys men's T-shirts because the seams are double stitched and she finds they hold up better than women's shirts. These days men's shirts come in a wide array of color.

KNOW YOUR FABRICS

We love fabrics made of natural fibers: linen, wool, and silk. God had a great idea when he created these fibers to clothe his children! Natural fibers breathe, they wear well, the fabric never goes out of style (although the garment may), and they hold their shape well.

Linen

Linen is a fiber made from a plant named flax. It has been used for clothing for thousands of years. Fabric made from linen threads is crisp and takes to tailoring very well. Linen garments are expensive if purchased from a regular department store. Garments made of linen will wrinkle when they are new. You have to get used to the fashionably wrinkled look. Linen fiber is often mixed with some man-made fiber to control wrinkling. Age, wearing the garment, and cleaning—whether washing or dry cleaning—eventually softens the fibers so that the garment does not wrinkle as much. That's when we like a linen garment best.

When you are purchasing a linen garment, consider it an investment that you will wear for several years. Sometimes it helps us justify the increased expense of a high-quality garment if we divide the cost of the garment by the number of years we plan to wear it. Then we will see that twenty dollars a year for five years isn't so much after all. If you are used to buying trendy, inexpensive clothes that you plan to wear only one year, buying higher-priced quality clothes for longevity might be something you have to think about. However, if you can find a new or almost new garment at a yard sale or thrift shop, then you are way ahead of the game.

Wool

If you can wear wool next to your skin, you are fortunate. Wool is a wonder fabric. It can be spun to be heavy enough for coats or fine enough for draped dresses and skirts. It's hard to beat the durability of a good wool gabardine fabric.

Wool is warm. It holds in body heat because it is dense and has air pockets that hold the warmth. Wool is warm even when wet. We do not recommend wearing wet wool, but if you get caught in a storm in a wool sweater, you have a better chance of avoiding hypothermia than if you were out in a man-made fiber.

100

When Gwen's children were small and the family did a lot of hiking in the mountains, a wool sweater was mandatory equipment, even in summer. Wool takes tailoring beautifully. Sleeves can be steamed and shaped to almost take a body's form. It will pleat or gather and can be rolled back to make an elegant collar. A well-tailored wool suit speaks quality loudly. No wonder our world leaders' suits are constructed of wool.

The problem with wool, as you may already know, is that it can be itchy. Some people cannot wear it. Collared shirts or scarves can keep a wool jacket from irritating your neck. Lining the garment helps, and lining also helps the garment hold its shape. Some wool will bag at the knees and where you sit. These days wool is often combined with man-made fibers for durability, comfort, ease of care, and to prevent stretching, but some of the flexibility and shapeability of the garment is lost when man-made fibers are added.

Watch for real wool garments when shoestring shopping. There seem to be a lot of them out there because they last forever. We suspect that people get tired of the garments long before they wear out, and that's why you find them in second-hand and consignment shops.

Silk

Silk is a luxurious fiber that can be spun to be anything from sheer to nubby and everything in between. Silk takes dye beautifully, and only on silk can certain colors be achieved. Anything with silk in it has breathability. Many people think silk is a cool fabric when indeed it can be very warm. Skiers know this and wear silk underwear under their ski outfits.

Silk can be washed in mild soap and cool water. But for longevity of color and because it is difficult to get all the wrinkles out of silk, you might want to send your silks to the dry cleaners. Take that into consideration when shoestring shopping because it adds to the total cost of a garment. Some silks are textured or prewrinkled. If you like that look, then buy away, because these silks are easy to wash, hang to dry, and are ready to wear again.

If you are unsure whether a silky garment is made of silk or of polyester, run your fingers over the fabric. If it feels like it is trying to cling to your fingers, it is real silk. Acetate, polyester, and other man-made fabrics may look a lot like silk, but they are very slick, while silk has an almost tacky feel to it.

Once we found it difficult to find silk in shoestring places, but now we find lots of it out there. Gwen has a classically styled red silk dress she has worn the last eleven summers. It still looks great and stylish.

Drawing the Line

Each person must decide how much shoestring shopping she wants to do. Even though you may find quality garments of all kinds, you may be more comfortable buying some of your garments at regular stores on sale or at outlet stores. Where is the line? Do you draw the line at buying used shoes? Would you ever consider buying used nightwear? Underwear? Only you can decide that for yourself.

We would encourage you to buy used "dry-clean only" clothing only if it has been cleaned, for several reasons. One is, of course, that you don't want to wear another person's dirty clothing. The second is that if you must have a garment dry-cleaned the minute you buy it, are you truly saving? The answer might be yes, but do take it into consideration.

Those are the basics of shopping for quality clothing, whether you find it on sale, in outlets, or at garage sales, consignment shops, and thrift shops. Use these tools and standards to assure you take home quality.

SHOESTRING TIPS

1. Spend time in clothing stores where you cannot possibly afford so much as a sock. There you can study and soak in the look and feel of quality.

2. Try on clothing in those stores to get an idea of how things should fit and look.

3. Do not be afraid to handle expensive clothing (with clean hands) to learn how it feels and how it is made.

4. Put the bulk of your clothing dollars into basic styles that will last for years and can be transformed with accessories.

5. Check the labels in clothing at shoestring places to find your favorite quality manufacturers and designers.

6. Remember that no matter how little something costs, if it doesn't fit properly, it is not a good investment.

7. Be careful with white pants. If they are not thick enough, you may as well wear nothing! Always wear properly fitting skin-tone briefs underneath. We have seen women and girls wearing skin-tight white stretch pants that showed every bulge, dimple, and panty design and color, and also how the bikini panties rode up one cheek.

SIX

THE HUNT IS ON

Warning: The hunt for clothing bargains is addictive. Gwen came around a corner in a favorite thrift store and there stood a friend in a mink jacket. Now this friend shopped only at the very best places in town and wore expensive, elegant clothing. Gwen could not imagine what she was doing here in a fur coat.

"Look what I found," she bubbled. "A mink jacket!"

"You found that here?" Gwen asked, incredulous both that her friend was here and that she had found something so beautiful.

"Yes, and it's only ninety-five dollars. Do you think I could get it for less?"

"Wouldn't hurt to try. What are you doing here?"

"I came with a friend. I've never been here before, but this is fun."

She's been bitten by the thrifting bug, Gwen thought. Her friend made an offer and it was accepted—a mink jacket for seventy-five dollars!

In a land of affluence where we produce way too much stuff, you can get what your family needs for far less than you would expect. The trick is to learn to plan ahead, be patient, and wait for the right item to present itself at a reduced price.

Right now a local Goodwill in Gwen's town has about thirty of the most beautiful wedding gowns you've ever laid eyes on. Each one of them is under fifty dollars. At a regular source these would cost hundreds of dollars or more.

A local discount shoe store went out of business and marked down their already discounted name-brand shoes 50 to 75 percent. Gwen bought two pair at this discount, and then a few weeks later, when closure was imminent and shoes were going for five dollars to ten dollars a pair, she bought two more pairs. She is well stocked with classic, simple, name-brand shoes that will still be in style ten years from now.

Before you rush out the door in search of terrific deals, let's go through a few pointers about smart shopping. These ideas will work for any kind of shopping but we will look at them with clothing in mind.

SMART SHOPPING

Like most things in life, it pays to be prepared. Preparation for shopping will take a little time and thought. So that you know a good price when you see one, study catalogs, read ads in your newspaper, and even do some window-shopping. Now, about that shopping trip:

First, decide where you will shop. From your newspaper you can learn where sales are for things on your list (we'll get to lists next). Read the classified ads if it is yard and garage sale season in your part of the country. The yellow pages of your phone book will help you find thrift stores, clearance places, and outlet stores. Find out the hours and days they are open. Use a map of your city to plan a good route for hitting all the places you want to visit.

Second, make a list and check it twice. We keep small notebooks in our purses for this. List needs for any gift giving you know is coming up (Christmas happens every year, as do birthdays and anniversaries), clothing for the next season, and any other purchases you need to make. You will need to include sizes, colors, fabric swatches, and measurements. Before Jo shops for a skirt for Anna at thrift stores, she measures the waistband of a skirt that fits Anna and writes that measurement down. If she finds a skirt that does not have a size tag in it, she can measure the waist to see if it is the right size. Jo even measures the waists of skirts with size tags in them because they vary so widely. Make notes on newspaper ads so you will not forget to check those stores for sale items.

Third, dress right. Wear comfortable walking shoes. If you plan to try on skirts or dresses, wear or bring hose so you will get a better idea of what the garment will look like when you are actually wearing it. No dress looks spiffy with athletic socks. Wear comfortable clothing that is easy to get on and off if you are shopping for yourself. You can either carry a very small purse to lighten your load, or a large one that will hold snacks and small purchases as well. Be sure to pack a small retractable tape measure and that all-important list.

Fourth, plan your budget. Decide how much you can spend. On that list you made, write down next to each item how much you want to spend on it. Do not forget to include an allowance for lunch or snacks in your budgeted shopping money unless you intend to pack your own. You will need to take a break from the exhausting job of shopping now and then, and you will get hungry. Is the car's gas tank full? That may have to be part of your planned spending as well.

Decide how you will pay for your purchase so that you will not go over your budget. Using cash is a surefire way to limit spending—no cheating at the ATM, though. Many yard sales do not take checks, but most stores do. Be sure to subtract each check to keep track of your spending. Remember, if you use a credit card, you must fully pay the statement each month to keep from paying interest. Those credit card bills can grow so fast, so easily. Keep a running total somehow to prevent overspending. Jo subtracts her Visa purchases from her checkbook balance so she can keep track of the total she spends, and then the money is already subtracted when it is time to pay the Visa bill. Only you know if you can trust yourself to use a credit card. If you have trouble handling credit responsibly, we recommend that you turn to Mary Hunt's *Cheapskate Monthly* newsletter for advice.

Let's take a look at several of the places you might shop for inexpensive, quality clothing.

GARAGE SALES

Cruisin' garage sales (or yard sales, or whatever you call them in your part of the country) is the perfect activity to do with a friend. We strongly suggest you not shop for clothing alone at these sales. A friend will help you find things and think through whether something is a wise purchase or not. A friend can help you inspect each garment. And you can help your friend. One of you can drive while the other navigates and looks for unadvertised yard sales along the way. And having a friend along is just more fun.

First scour the newspaper classified ads for sales and plan an efficient route. Bring along a map of your city. Taking a lunch is a good idea. Not only do you not literally "eat up" your savings at a restaurant, but you can also save a lot of time by eating in the car or at a park along the way. That means more time for sales. Jo and her yard sale shopping buddy, Vickie, take turns driving and packing lunches.

You can find all kinds of clothing at garage sales, but the best buys are probably accessories and kids' clothing. Since kids grow so fast and their clothing is generally well made, you can often find wonderful bargains. Oshkosh overalls and pants for kids seem to never wear out.

In the thrill of finding things so cheap, do not forget to exercise the same care you would if you were spending a great deal more. When you find that adorable little top for your young daughter, take it into the light and inspect it. Are there any rips or tears? Are there stains? Will those stains come out, or are they in a place that can be covered with a decorative patch or trim? Does the garment look worn? There will be a lot of yard sales, so you can afford to be picky.

Do not buy used shoes for your kids. Shoes take the shape of the wearer's feet, so unless the shoes are brand new and a perfect fit, you will condemn your kids to literally "walking in someone else's shoes" and perhaps acquiring foot and leg problems. Dress shoes and snow boots that are worn infrequently may be the exceptions.

If you sew, watch for items like fabric, buttons, zippers, trim, and sewing supplies. These items can be expensive in retail stores. If you have a small supply of these items on hand, it saves you money as well as the time it would take to get to a store and purchase them. But don't accumulate too much sewing stuff, especially fabric, because fabric styles do change. Good bets are blue denim and white cottons. Prints go out of style quickly, and double knits have gone out of style to stay. Polyesters are also passé.

THRIFT SHOPS

Gwen thought she knew everything there was to know about shopping in thrift stores until recently. She was in Seattle visiting her daughter and had a couple of extra hours on her way to an appointment. She stopped at the main headquarters of a large thrift store chain and discovered that this store had an outlet center. She watched as a forklift moved five four-foot square bales into the outlet.

Her curiosity was piqued, so she went inside and found customers eagerly pawing through clothing and fabric goods piled on tables. She approached the nearest table and began to paw too.

She began checking labels. They were brand names: Eddie Bauer, Nordstrom, Jaeger, J. G. Hook, and so on. Some of the garments were obviously used, but many looked brand new. She found a big, fluffy mint-green terry bathrobe in perfect condition. Next she found two towels—brand new—then a throw rug and a fitted queen-sized sheet, all in perfect condition. All of these finds were weighed and sold for ninety-nine cents per pound.

On another table, garments actually had prices on them. They were forty-nine cents for any item on the table. She bought a brand-new sweater with a car pattern woven into it for her five-year-old great-nephew. She bought a Pacific Trail jacket for herself. Her total bill was nine dollars.

What's the explanation for this "steal"? Seattle is headquarters to Nordstrom stores, and with their amazing "no questions asked" return policy, they have to dispose of returns someplace. The same would go for Eddie Bauer and other manufacturers in that area. Gwen suspects that returns are bundled into bales and sold to thrift outlets.

Thrift stores have unique "personalities"—different stores carry different kinds of merchandise. Some have racks of designer clothes. Some even have boutique areas. Some sell lots of brand-new clothing, tags still in place. Some have terrible clothing but great appliances. Learn which shops carry what you are looking for. Then ask when the shops put out new merchandise.

Shops run by charity organizations that receive donations from people with higher incomes will tend to have better quality. Shops located in upscale neighborhoods will also have a better selection. Shops in areas where clothing is manufactured will sometimes carry a manufacturer's overruns.

Know your brand names and labels. As we have said before, browsing in quality department stores will help you recognize brand names and excellent quality as well as style. You cannot afford to buy a garment at a thrift shop if it is already out of style. That's why classics are such good purchases. A crew neck Shetland wool sweater has been in style for decades and will continue to be so. A straight, lined wool skirt in a neutral color will never go out of style. A cable-knit cardigan will still be stylish ten years from now. Good leather belts are a wise investment—especially when you only pay a couple of dollars for them.

OUTLET MALLS

The difference between outlet malls and "real" factory outlets is great. Outlet malls have become big business. They are often located in out-of-the-way places to keep the cost of doing business as low as possible. We have found, however, that prices in outlet malls are only marginally better than in retail stores and sometimes no better at all than sale prices at department stores and regular malls. When you add in the time needed to reach an outlet mall, the distance traveled, and the fact that you will probably have to eat at least one meal away from home, you might not be saving as much as you think.

However, when an outlet mall is moving last season's inventory, you can find some real bargains. The shops in an outlet mall are generally small and have little storage. Therefore they must clear out last season's stock. Prices are sometimes cut as much as 70 percent.

It's about as much fun to buy winter sweaters on a hot summer day as it is to buy short-sleeved T-shirts on a cold winter day. But winter comes around again every year and so does summer. Your family will need clothes next season as well as this one. So think ahead when shopping outlet malls and indeed all other sources as well. Shoestring budgets require planning ahead.

If you really want to take advantage of an outlet mall, go there planning to do a season's worth of shopping at one time. Because you will find everything from tools to underwear outlets in one place, you can do a lot of shopping in a day. Plan to make it an all-day outing and either take a lunch or buy one in the food shops of the mall. Go armed with your notebook of sizes, family needs, household needs, and color preferences (see chart on page 121).

REAL FACTORY OUTLETS

The difference between a shopping mall outlet and a "real" factory outlet is that real factory outlets are attached to the factory where the items being sold are made. This is where the manufacturer gets rid of overruns, mistakes, and bits and pieces of things used to make their product. For example:

- Pendleton Woolen Mills in Oregon sells garments, woolen fabric, blankets, zippers, buttons, and so forth.

- Sportscaster manufactures jackets in Seattle. In the basement you can buy ski clothes, jackets, and coats as well as fiberfill, outdoor fabrics, zippers, and buttons.

- The Jessica McClintock factory outlet in San Francisco sells their entire line of beautiful dress-up garments at one-third to one-half off. Here too you can buy lace, zippers, fabrics, and a host of other items used in the construction of that line of clothing.

While it isn't economical to travel across the country to shop for clothing at one of these "real" factory outlets, keep your eyes open when you are traveling. If you hear of a factory store, you may find it worth your time to go a bit out of your way to see what is there. Think of it as a serendipitous adventure.

Be careful to inspect garments in these shops to make sure they do not have obvious mistakes. Some mistakes are so miniscule that no will notice them and you can live with them, but if a piece of the front has been sewn wrong side out, that's a big problem.

Check for mistakes in print, threads missing from a woven plaid, flaws in the fabric, and unmatched plaid. Ask the clerk to show you the flaw in a garment marked "seconds" before deciding whether to purchase the item.

When Gwen travels across a state line by car, she stops at the visitors' welcome center where she often finds pamphlets listing outlet sources in the state. In Massachusetts she discovered the real factory outlets in Fall River, southwest of Boston. She was intrigued by the name of one outlet—"Nobody's Perfect"—where ladies', men's, and children's clothing as well as accessories from well-known specialty and department stores are sold at 40 to 80 percent off.

CONSIGNMENT SHOPS

Another source of good clothing is consignment shops. We have never seen a consignment shop exclusively for men's clothing but we have found plenty that carry women's and children's clothing. The prices in consignment shops tend to be a little higher than at thrift stores or other shoestring sources because the shop must make a small profit on every garment sold in order to stay in business. However, the upside is that there are strict rules for what such shops will carry. Clothing must be fairly up-to-date, clean, mended, hanging on a hanger, and ready to wear. One advantage in buying used clothing at a consignment shop rather than at a thrift store is that it is in such great condition when purchased. Clothing you buy at a thrift shop must be dry-cleaned or laundered before it can be worn because all garments are sold "as is."

Consignment shops carry better dresses, suits, and coats and a good assortment of dress-up clothing. They also carry handbags, shoes, jewelry, and other accessories. We women are a fickle lot when it comes to what we like and want. Those who can afford to change their minds and buy new clothing or accessories have to do something with cast-off clothing. Some of us choose to sell our castoffs in shops like these. Jo regularly buys and sells her clothing at her nearby neighborhood consignment shop.

VINTAGE SHOPPING ALONG MEMORY LANE

Vintage shopping might be called "shopping along memory lane." It has become a sizeable industry in this country. You can find vintage clothing shops in most towns. While this style of dressing is not for everyone, some people really like buying older clothing. Years ago clothing was made with great care and attention to detail. People did not buy clothing just to throw it out and buy more the next season. They bought clothing to last many years or even to hand down to the next generation.

In a vintage clothing shop, the Romantic will find elegant, lacy, exquisite dresses unlike anything made today. A vintage clothing shop Jo enjoys visiting has a selection of antique wedding dresses, suits, evening gowns, undergarments, children's dresses, beaded bags, elegant gloves, hats, handkerchiefs, jewelry, and hair ornaments. A Romantic could compile an entire outfit in this shop.

These shops also carry things from every decade up to the seventies. We find Jackie Kennedy suits and pillbox hats. We have laughed at granny gowns, which were popular in the sixties. We are sure some of the clothing came straight from Aunt

Martha's closet or was sent to the shop when some dear old relative died.

An Artsy-Creative or High Fashion–Dramatic person may find just the right thing among these memorable garments. You may look perfect wearing some of the art deco items, one-of-a-kind accessories, and fur coats found in these shops.

Vintage shops carry things that have been out of style so long that they are back in style again. Who would have ever thought that the sweater set would come back? Sixties fashions have also come back in style. Bell-bottoms, anyone?

You may have your own vintage clothing shop in an attic. Perhaps you could search your own storage areas for boxes of clothing you have put away. Or see if your mother or other relatives have packed away some vintage clothing. Go through their boxes. You might just find a fabulous sweater set. Jo owns two flashy brooches that were passed on to her from her Grandma Pulsipher many years ago. They jazz up some of Jo's coats and blazers.

Watch for the "little black dress" that has never gone out of style. Make sure that the fabric has not turned shiny, especially where the wearer sits. Look for jewelry, a lace shawl, jackets, and scarves to accessorize your little black dress.

No matter what your style, these vintage stores can be just the place for you to find unique clothing that is truly you. And they are fun to shop in even if you never buy a thing.

DISCOUNT STORES

Working in the book industry, Gwen has learned that the merchandise sold to large chains of discount stores is the same merchandise sold to specialty shops. That goes for clothing as well. Simple, everyday clothing is sold to discount stores in huge quantities and at great discounts and is then resold to the customer at excellent prices. T-shirts, underwear, socks, jeans, shorts, and nightwear are among some of the best bargains.

Of course, the time to get the big bargains is at the change of the seasons. Look for summer clothing to go on sale right after July 4. (Check out our handy chart at the end of this chapter for more examples.) When the selling seasons change, the theme in many discount stores might well be, "round 'em up, move 'em out!" You will be the beneficiary of the store's need to purge. Arrive early and shop smart.

Catalog and Online Shopping

There are two shopping options that do not require leaving the comfort of your own home. Catalog and online shopping grow in popularity every year. As with any other shopping, be careful. It is even more important to know good quality and good prices when you shop this way. Be sure to add the price of shipping and handling to the cost of anything you buy.

Catalog Shopping

Gwen grew up in a little town in Montana, far away from any major shopping area. Her hometown had a couple of stores that sold clothing and one store that actually sold *quality* clothing, and that was about it. This tiny town was thirty-five miles from the nearest town where any significant shopping could be done. Catalogs were often the shopping source for back-to-school, Christmas, and other general shopping.

The arrival of the Sears, Roebuck and Co. and Montgomery Wards Christmas catalogs was cause for a huge celebration. Gwen would spend hours pouring over those "wish books."

The L. L. Bean catalog was popular with all the hunters and fishermen who lived in Montana. This was their source for shoes called "pacs." A pac is a one-piece rubber shoe attached to a lace-up leather upper that has been waterproofed. With a sheep-skin liner, pacs are about as warm and comfortable as any shoe can be. Hunters also found their favorite red-and-black plaid woolen coats and caps in the L. L. Bean catalog. Fishermen found all their hats and other clothing accouterments in this catalog. Gwen recalls her father studying his catalog while sitting in his old easy chair, feet propped up, in front of a fire. Such are the joys of catalog shopping.

Of course there is a downside to catalog shopping as well. If you get clothing that is not right for you or a family member because of size, color, or personal preference, your purchases must be returned. That can be a time-consuming hassle. So you really must know yourself and your family members' tastes, preferences, and sizes when ordering from a catalog.

The other downside is that you are not able to inspect, feel, and try on the clothing. What looks like a million dollars on a model may be made of cheap fabric or have shoddy workmanship or a scanty cut when it arrives in the mail. Remember that unless you are built like a model, the clothing will look a lot different on you than it does on a model. The right clothing can do a lot to make us look our best, but it cannot turn Jo, who is five-foot-six-inches tall with bulges where she does not want them, into a five-foot-ten-inch, long-legged, skinny beauty. She will be disappointed every time!

If you enjoy catalog shopping or wish to try it, you can get on catalog mailing lists easily. Many popular magazines have a regular feature in the back that lists all kinds of catalogs. They often have a card with little numbers on it that correspond to the three-inch ads in the magazine. Pick a couple of catalogs that feature what you like or wish for, fill out the card, and in a few weeks you will receive your catalogs. But be warned that those catalogs will sell their mailing lists to other companies, so before you know it, you will receive a plethora of catalogs. They will keep coming whether you buy anything or not, so don't feel you must buy something. Catalogs make it easier to do comparison shopping. You can also "shop" at home with a family member to find out their current tastes. Jo goes through the JCPenney catalog with her daughter and marks each clothing item with "yes" or "no" to learn what Anna likes. However you use your catalogs, always keep your budget in mind!

Online Shopping

You can spend money quickly and easily online. All you need is a credit card, Internet access, and a lack of self-control. Since we are shoestring shoppers, though, we will control ourselves and use the web to get great buys.

To find web sites that offer clothing, just type the keyword "clothing" into a search engine. You will get more options than you know what to do with. Narrow your search by being more specific or by searching for a particular company's web site.

Shop wisely. Know your size, what color and styles you want, and what you want to spend. Remember that you do not have to buy something the moment you see it. You can take some time to think about it and shop some more. This is not the last opportunity you will have. There will be other great offers in the future.

You might want to try using the Internet to hunt for used children's clothing as well. Search for the phrase "hand-me-down clothing" and see what comes up. We live in amazing times, don't we?

Since her schedule is so busy, Gwen has recently been enjoying a little online clothing shopping. It saved her a lot of time and energy! She was looking for work clothes and found three nice dresses in the jewel tones that are so becoming on her. All three totaled one hundred dollars. She likes dresses because they make mornings easier. No mixing or matching (or thinking!) first thing in the morning. She leaves some of the accessories—like pins and scarves—attached to her dresses if she plans to wear them again before sending them to the dry cleaner or washing them. That eliminates searching for the right accessories before she is feeling fully awake.

CARRY A NOTEBOOK

Smart shoestring shoppers carry a notebook. Here's an idea of what a page of your notebook might look like. (See chart on page 121. This chart may be photocopied.) Don't go shopping without your chart. Fill it in and update it frequently (kids grow fast and their sizes change). Since time is money, you can't waste time any more than you can waste money. And you don't have to—just go prepared, think about what you are doing, and resist giving in to whims. If you have a child who is picky about what he or she wears, make a date to go shopping with that child and persevere until that child has what is needed for the next season. Teens have their own ideas about what's "cool," so if you don't want to waste time returning clothing to the store (sometimes you can't return sale clothing), take the teen along. When shopping means they get new clothes, most teens are willing to go along.

Those with picky teens must remember that you want them to grow up to be independent, and their choices in clothing are one of the first places teens can begin to differentiate between themselves and their parents. While you may hate the way they look for a few years, it's a fairly safe place for them to exercise their personality and independence.

BEST TIMES TO BUY

This list will help you know when to look for certain kinds of clothing on sale.

January

Costume jewelry	Infant wear
Dresses	Men's clothing
Furs	Shoes
Handbags	Sportswear
Men's hats	

February
Women's hats
Sportswear

Men's shirts

March
Spring clothing
Winter coats

Boys' and girls' shoes

April
Women's and children's coats
Dresses
Women's hats

Housecoats
Infant wear
Men's and boys' suits

May
Handbags
Housecoats

Lingerie

June
Dresses
Housecoats

Summer clothes and fabrics

July
Bathing suits
Children's clothing
Children's hats
Infant wear

Lingerie
Men's shirts
Shoes
Sportswear

August
Bathing suits
Coats
Furs

Men's clothing
School clothes

September
Not much!

October
Housecoats

School clothes

Name	Color preference	Shirt size/ needs	Skirt or pants size/ needs	Shoe size/ needs	Socks styles/ needs	Dress size/needs (females)	Jacket size/ needs

November
Children's clothing   Dresses
Women's and children's coats   Housecoats

December
Children's clothing   Children's hats
Women's and children's coats

Let the shopping begin!

SHOESTRING TIPS

1. Take a ten-dollar bill to a thrift store and see how many truly useful, needed, and well-made things you can buy with it.

2. Shop at shoestring places for what you need before going to retail stores.

3. For special occasions, check out consignment shops that sell very dressy garments. Most glittery, spangled, satin, and bowed dresses are only worn once or twice before they are no longer useful to the owners.

4. Try shopping online. A site called "Chic Simple" on AOL's shopping web site shows you the basic pieces for a casual Friday look or a more formal office attire look. Check prices carefully before you buy online. Also check the return policies of the companies. Nothing is more expensive than buying something that does not work and then not being able to return it.

5. Coordinate and communicate with your friends so you can be on the lookout for each other. Jo's friend Vickie knew that Jo was looking for a certain kind of jacket and found it for her at a ninety-nine cent sale at a thrift store. Jo is keeping her eye out for a pair of Lee jeans, size 8, that a friend needs.

6. Buy only what you need. Save your money for those things.

7. Be picky.

8. Carry a retractable measuring tape.

9. Do not shop when you are hurried, hungry, tired, ill, or stressed. You will not make the best decisions.

10. When shopping with a friend, divide and conquer: "You check the kids' clothes while I check out the shoes."

11. Quit shopping when you get too tired to inspect each purchase thoroughly or when you just want to go home.

12. Have fun!

SEVEN

TO KEEP OR NOT TO KEEP, THAT IS THE QUESTION

Sally was on a rampage. Her family had to defend every piece of clothing they wanted to keep or Sally would ruthlessly snatch it away. She had good reasons, of course.

First of all, her family had a habit of growing emotionally attached to things they could no longer wear. This made their closets and dresser drawers impossible to keep tidy.

Second, it was March. Her church held a clothing exchange that month. Sally wanted to donate a lot to the clothing exchange, and she also planned to take advantage of the opportunity to get free clothing for her family. But first she had to go through everyone's closets to see what was there. Sally ruthlessly sorted each family member's clothing into five piles: discard, laundry, restyle, mend, and keep.

The discard pile grew fast. Sally's green dress, an outgrown suit, that blouse like Natasha's, the skirt that made her hips look big, the dress with an immodestly short hemline, and the jacket in a bold print all landed in the discard pile. Ted's leisure suit (maybe the church drama department could use it for their costume collection), Bruce's jeans that hadn't fit for six weeks, and some of Spacy's outgrown clothing joined the pile.

It was embarrassing to Sally that she even needed to make a laundry pile. But she found dirty clothing hiding in everyone's closets! Bruce was the worst offender. Ted was also a major donor of soiled clothing with several food-spotted ties, a blazer, and a sweater that all needed dry cleaning. The laundry room was a mess now, with new piles of laundry everywhere, and a big pile of clothing waited by the back door to be taken to Do-It-Cheap Dry Cleaners.

In the restyle pile were things that were outdated or no longer fit but could be salvaged with a little sewing. One pair of Sally's pants has hopelessly wide legs. She considers them for a moment, then sees that the knees and seat are worn. She tosses them onto the discard pile. There are a couple of blouses with silly ruffles. They look like they could be redeemed if she removed the ruffles. Ted has a couple of pairs of wool dress slacks collecting dust on his side of the closet. He admits that they are a bit snug around the waist. Sally is sure she can let them out enough to make them comfortable again.

The mending pile becomes larger as Sally inspects all the clothing her family wants to keep. Many garments have been out of circulation due to missing buttons, sagging hems, and split seams. Sally vows to herself that she will make the mending pile a priority next week.

The piles of clothing the family will keep are returned to the closets. Those closets will need organizing later. (You can read about how to do that in chapter 10 in this book.)

126

Sally redirects her attention to the huge discard pile. She gives each item one more look. Is anything worth restyling? Nope. Two pairs of jeans are so frayed they just can't be salvaged. They land in the trash. While inspecting those wide-legged pants, Sally finds an earring she has been missing for a few years in a pocket! Eventually the discarded clothing is neatly folded and put into boxes headed for the clothing exchange.

The church clothing exchange began a few years ago as a kids' clothing exchange. A men's tie exchange was begun by some enterprising men. Then someone got the idea of combining the two events and including clothing and accessories for the whole family.

Here's how the event works. For a day or two before the exchange, a large room is reserved for people to drop off their unwanted clothing. Volunteers organize the clothing as it arrives in the following way:

- Menswear is on one side with a table for sweaters, sweats, and accessories, racks of hanging clothing, and a special spot for all those ties.

- Ladies' wear, the largest area, is organized with different racks for dresses, skirts, pants, and tops and tables full of folded sweaters and accessories.

- Boys' and girls' clothing is hung separately.

- Baby clothing is placed on tables that are labeled according to size.

Large signs on racks and tables clearly lead people to what they want. By the end of the drop-off period, the place looks like a very nice thrift store.

The next day the "store" is open for a few hours. Everybody from the church and their friends are welcome to come and take whatever they find that they need. No money is exchanged.

Sally's family will shop only for those things they need. They will take only what fits, looks good on them, and is truly needed. They do not want to be greedy or grabby.

At the end of the day, the hangers and racks are stored for the next exchange. The leftover clothing is given to local charities. The baby clothing goes to the local pregnancy center. Some clothing may be given to missions projects.

Sally has been excited about the exchange since she read about it the first time in the church bulletin. Not only is she donating her family's discards, but she has also volunteered to spend a few hours organizing the clothing as it comes in. She is glad that other families can benefit from her hand-me-downs. She will also form some lasting friendships with the other church members who volunteer that day.

WHY WEAR HAND-ME-DOWNS?

When we add clothing a family to all the other things in our budgets, it gets to be quite a balancing act. Only so much money comes through the family bank account each month. The point of a budget is to have priorities for where the money will be spent. What is important to your family?

For most of us, wearing nice clothing is not what we remember most fondly about our childhood. Family vacations, special occasions, and much-anticipated events often make up our fond childhood memories. On the other hand, some of us have painful childhood memories of not being able to dress as nicely as others. Our parents either could not afford to clothe us the way we wanted to be clothed or did not consider it necessary to do so.

A tried-and-true method of reducing the clothing budget is the practice of handing down clothes. Handing down can take place within a family or extended family, within the church family, and with neighbors. However it is accomplished, it is usually very much appreciated by all involved.

When Gwen was growing up, she occasionally received boxes of clothing from a young woman who was an only child. Getting a box from that source was truly an adventure because that little girl's parents bought her only the best. Very early on, Gwen began devising ways to make the handed down clothing fit her style. She took two-piece outfits apart and wore the parts with clothing she already had in her closets. She added accessories. She learned her shoestring clothing skills early in life!

Jo's kids have always worn hand-me-downs. They realize that the budget can stretch only so far. They also realize that if they do not spend too much on clothing, the family can go out to eat occasionally, attend a baseball game, save for a vacation, or simply enjoy an impromptu visit to their favorite ice cream parlor.

At first the hand-me-downs came from a family member and some friends at church. Then Jo got brave and asked people if they wanted her hand-me-downs. That led to others in her circle of friends doing the same for her. Her last neighborhood had a whole system of passing hand-me-downs between all the mothers of little boys and girls on the block. Some little dresses went through all five families in the "system" before being sent out of the neighborhood. Sometimes Anna could hardly wait for her slightly older and bigger friend to grow out of a cute and desirable outfit so that she could have her turn wearing it.

There are some hand-me-downs we simply would not consider wearing, regardless of who handed them down, how nice they are, or what condition they are in. Underwear falls in that category. We buy underwear and socks in bulk at discount stores. Jo has tricks for keeping three guys' underwear and socks separate and easy to identify when it is time to sort laundry. The whole family knows the tricks because the whole family shares the responsibilities of doing laundry. Jo's system does not involve writing anyone's name or initials anywhere or doing any sewing.

That would be too much work and the clothes would still be hard to identify with a quick, casual glance.

The "brief" trick: Each guy in the family wears a different brand of briefs. These brands are easily identifiable by the brand names and colored threads that are woven into the waistbands. Jo began this method many years ago, when her boys were quite young. She had trouble figuring out whose underwear was whose. Sometimes the tags identifying the size would fade or come off entirely after several washings. After using her brand method of sorting for several years, all the guys know who wears what brand and can help to keep briefs sorted.

Here's Jo's athletic sock trick: Each of the guys likes a different sock style. Even Mom and Anna have distinctive styles so the whole sorting game is easy. Socks are all bought in big packs of six at a discount store, making it easy to stock up and to replace them. At laundry sorting time, everyone knows that Dad gets the boring plain white ones, Josh gets the ones with a colorful stripe, Jon's are heavily ribbed, Mom's are short, and Anna's are more like anklets. A family member can change his preferred style of socks at any time—he just cannot choose one that somebody else is currently using.

Other hand-me-downs besides underwear come into a household but are not usable. Jo's daughter Anna has definite ideas about what styles she will wear, what colors she likes, and what is comfortable. Jo does not keep the things Anna doesn't like. She also does not keep clothing that is beyond repair or badly stained. Plus, not everything will fit, be modest, or be in style.

The Janssen boys rarely receive hand-me-downs now that they are adult sized. However, once in a while an adult male friend passes on items that he has grown out of. Josh enjoys wearing the camouflage jacket a friend gave him. Dad's dress shirts, socks, and ties come in handy and sometimes take up permanent residence in one of the boys' closets.

Keeping something in a child's closet that he or she has rejected is pointless. The rejects and clothing Anna has grown out of go to some friends with three daughters who are smaller than Anna. Jo's boys wear out their clothes before they grow out of them nowadays, but the few things that do survive get passed along to friends or end up in the church clothing exchange. It is important to pass on the blessing of hand-me-downs. It truly is more blessed and fun to give than to receive.

As we mentioned above, some hand-me-downs are worn, torn, or stained beyond hope. However, some of those items may still be redeemable with a little imagination.

Before deciding whether or not to try to fix a garment, analyze it carefully. Will the garment really be worn? Does it fit perfectly? Is it becoming? Will another coordinating garment have to be purchased to make it work in the wardrobe? Is it up-to-date? Is it faded? Is it of good quality? Does the future wearer really like and want it? You do not want to put effort, time, and even a little money into something that isn't going to be worn or won't look great when it is fixed.

Now look at what is wrong with the garment. How bad is it? Some problems can be creatively hidden or fixed. Some cannot. Some stains cannot be removed, but you may be able to hide them. Some rips and tears may be too large to mend unobtrusively. Tears in seams can usually be easily mended. Missing buttons can be replaced. Broken zippers can be replaced as well. Maybe it only needs to be washed, starched, and ironed. With a good idea of what you are capable of and what you are willing to try, decide if this fix-it project is worth tackling or not. If it won't cost anything to try and you have the time and tools, go for it. You do not have much to lose. If it is out of your mending comfort zone and ability level and will cost money to repair, give it a second thought.

Perhaps the hand-me-down just needs a little updating. Changing decorative details can update or cheer up an outfit.

This could be as simple as changing the buttons. Trims can be removed, changed, or added. We cover that in chapter 8.

The length of shorts, slacks, jackets, sleeves, and tops vary as styles change. It doesn't take much to shorten these things, but it can be next to impossible to lengthen them. They may have worn creases or lack enough hem allowance to allow lengthening. Are you willing to tackle this? Again, we give you more on this in chapter 8.

People who give us hand-me-downs may not share our coloring. Consequently, what looked terrific on the blond neighbor kids may not be very becoming on our dark-haired children.

We can always dye things. If the garment isn't worn near the face, such as pants or skirts, we can still use it by wearing a becoming color on top. So when a winter person receives a brown pair of pants, he can wear a white top and still look great. Sweaters, jumpers, vests, overalls, and sweatshirts can go over shirts that are not the right color. Just make sure the separate items do not clash! However, unless you really need that garment that is the wrong color, we do not recommend cluttering your lives with things that do not coordinate with the rest of the wardrobe. Pass them on to someone who will look great in them.

KNOW WHAT YOU HAVE

You can't even begin to think about repairing and restyling your clothing or adding to your wardrobe until you find out what you already have. So the first thing to do is to take everything out of the closet and pile it somewhere—probably on a bed. Then give the closet a good cleaning and if it needs it some new paint, shelves, rods, hooks, hangers, and whatever it takes to make it work for you. Good closet organization will help you keep track of what you have (more about that later). You might want to give yourself a couple of days for this cleaning and sorting project the first time you do it. As you repeat this process on a regular seasonal cycle, it won't take as long, because you will have thinned your closet to have only those clothes that fit you well, please you, are flattering, and are in good repair. A working wardrobe!

Sort the clothing into categories. Make a pile of blouses and shirts, one of skirts, one of pants, one of dresses, one of suits or suit jackets. Don't forget your shoes. Sort them by usage: dress, play, and work. Sort scarves, ties, belts, and other accessory items as well.

We are not asking you to do anything we have not done ourselves. At the recent change of the season, Gwen pulled everything out of her closet and went to work sorting. Jo does this twice a year with each child, herself, and her husband. The next step is evaluating what we have.

Most of us have too many clothes in our closets that we are not wearing. Gwen will confess to that. Because she buys clothes cheaply, she easily accumulates too many. Her recent closet-sorting party led her to evaluate everything and thin out a huge bag of clothes that she still liked but for one reason or another had not worn in the last season or two. Out the door went the bag and off to a thrift shop to help someone who could be using the garments before they go completely out of style.

You are going to make five piles of clothing: discard, laundry, restyle, mend, and keep. Everything will go into one of those piles or back into your closet. So, pick up the first piece of clothing and ask yourself some questions that will help you evaluate each piece.

When was the last time this was worn? If the last time was more than a year ago, toss the garment in the discard pile.

Is it still liked? If the answer is "Yes, I like it, but I haven't worn it," be realistic and add it to the discard pile.

Was it a mistake in the first place? Sometimes we just have to cut our losses, admit our mistakes, and move on. The discard pile grows.

Is it great just the way it is? Is it in good repair? If the answer to these questions is yes, put the garment in the keep pile. Here's one piece of clothing you don't have to deal with because it is already wearable. If it needs repairing, put it in the mending pile. You will find help for your mending in the next chapter.

Does it fit, or am I waiting to lose ten pounds so that I can wear it? If it does not fit, put it in the discard pile now. By the time you lose weight, it will probably be out of style. It is easier to admit mistakes, thin your wardrobe, and let go of old favorites if you think about the person who will be getting the garments. Think how thrilled that person will be to have something new to wear right now. It could well be someone who really needs the over-flow of your closet. (We know of an organization that gives women a start in business by training them to have marketable skills and then providing them with a couple of suits for their interviews and beginning days of work. Look for an organization that is helping people either by giving them clothing or by sell-ing used clothing and using the proceeds to help others.) By the way, clothing that is too big looks just as bad as clothing that is too small. Discard it.

Is this garment of high enough quality to be worthy of renovation? If the answer is yes, the garment is added to the pile of clothing to be restyled. We will tell you how later.

Are the color and style flattering? If the answer is no, the gar-ment goes in the discard pile. Learn your best colors and stick to them (reread chapter 2).

Does it match anything I have, or do I have to buy more clothing to make it work in my wardrobe? If it truly suits you and the only rea-son it does not match anything in your wardrobe is because the rest of your wardrobe does not suit you, consider this item the beginning of your new clothing collection. However—and we have a feeling this is more likely—if nothing in your wardrobe matches what you are holding in your hand or if it just doesn't suit you, get rid of it.

Does the garment need washing or a trip to the cleaners? Dry cleaning is expensive and we encourage you not to have many garments that have to be dry cleaned. You will, however, always have a few garments that need it. If you can, wait for a discount coupon or special at the cleaners. Take your clothes at that time. You might be able to find a dry cleaner that does cleaning by the pound. Some of these establishments clean clothes but do not press them. If saving money is a key factor, consider doing your own pressing. If time is a factor, use a dry cleaner that will do it as part of the price.

Proceed through your wardrobe asking the questions above about every piece of clothing you own. Be ruthless. It only hurts for a little while, and afterward each member of your family will be so pleased with his or her efficient, working wardrobe.

You might want to salvage some of your castoffs that can be turned into cleaning rags. Gwen cuts up 100 percent cotton T-shirts when they have become too faded from washing or stained (from some of her shoestring decorating projects) and uses them for dishcloths and dusting rags. It doesn't make sense to her to throw them away and then turn around and buy dishcloths. She uses old sheets for drop cloths, for window cleaning, and as polishing rags. It's just another way to save money.

If giving your clothing away is just too painful, you can have a garage sale and sell your clothing, but don't expect to sell it all or to get much for what you do sell. As mentioned before, you can also sell good, clean used clothing at consignment shops where you share the profit with the shop owner. Check with your local consignment shop for rules, regulations, and the percentage you will get, and find out what happens to your clothing at the end of the allotted selling time. Use the proceeds to either buy other clothing or to get out of debt and free yourself financially.

The way you choose to get rid of clothing you are not using is up to you; the important thing is to get rid of it. You will probably have plenty left, and if you do not have plenty left, you will know what you need once you have thinned your closet. Then you can go out and buy those pieces that will make what's left work best. In Gwen's recent foray through her closet, she discovered she really doesn't have enough short-sleeved summer blouses. So she will concentrate on adding some that will work with the skirts and slacks she has kept.

If you are not sure about whether or not to discard an item, fold the clothing, put it in labeled boxes, and store the box in the garage for a while. If you haven't reclaimed a piece of clothing in a month or more, get rid of the whole box.

Put the dirty machine-washable clothing items in the wash. Then do all the hand washing at once.

Remember that pile of clothing that needs mending or restyling? We are going to tackle that in the next chapter. Few things give as much satisfaction as restoring a quality piece of clothing to active service by doing a little mending or restyling.

Shoestring Tips

1. Talk to your friends about trading hand-me-downs once or twice a year.

2. Begin a clothing exchange at your church or in your neighborhood.

3. If you really cannot use an item, pass it on.

4. Learn how to mend.

5. Press and spray starch cotton garments to make them look nicer. If you don't like the stiffness of starch in your clothes, at least use a spray-on fabric finish, available where you buy spray starch.

6. Always try clothing on; do not trust sizes on the tags.

7. Use the library to find entire books on removing stains from fabrics. Check one out to see if you can remove what looks like a hopeless stain. Look around the 648.1 section if your library uses the Dewey decimal system or TX324.C66 if your library uses the Library of Congress cataloging numbers.

8. When someone gives you hand-me-downs, do something nice for him or her. Bake cookies? Baby-sit? At least a thank-you note!

9. Organize hand-me-downs stored for future use according to sex, season, and size, marking boxes for easy identification later. A box's label might read, "Boys, summer, 4T."

10. Are some of the hand-me-downs good prospects for the dress-up and play make-believe trunk? Every kid loves to create pretend worlds. Costumes help. Keep a trunk of clothing and accessories gleaned from hand-me-downs just for play.

11. Businessmen can do a tie exchange as a fun way to get together for an evening and to get a "new" tie without spending a lot of money.

12. Clothing that came from a boy (like a shirt) can be made feminine for a girl with the addition of ruffled lace, bows, ribbons, and pretty patches.

13. Have a positive attitude about hand-me-downs. Isn't God good to give us all these clothes just when we needed them! Your children are watching you . . . and your thankful attitude!

EIGHT

It's Time to Mend Your Ways

Jo once made the mistake of trying to work part-time when all her kids were in school. Many mothers can successfully pull off the Super Mom trick. Jo could not. Things got left undone that her family had grown accustomed to having done—and that included the mending.

It wasn't a pretty sight. The pile of mending grew so fast that it became too depressing to even look at. Al was wearing a raincoat with buttons hanging on by mere threads and then falling off altogether. The kids couldn't live without their favorite pants, so they would keep wearing them even though the split in the seams got bigger and bigger. Like we said, it wasn't a pretty sight.

Jo eventually realized her mistake and quit working outside the home. By then, though, she had spent her hard-earned money replacing clothes she could have simply mended if she had not been so tired.

Would your family have more clothes if you did some mending? Well, let's get to it before your kids grow out of those clothes and that jacket with the missing button goes out of style!

When it comes to mending, there's a simple rule that most of us, like Jo for a while, do not follow very well. This rule will ensure a wardrobe that works: Do not put anything away that is not perfectly ready to wear. That means no stockings with runs put back in the drawer. No garments with loose or completely detached buttons rehung in the closet. No garments with hems that are falling out put away. No garments with split seams or malfunctioning zippers left to be grabbed sometime when you are in a terrible hurry and do not have the patience for much frustration.

If you sew, you can take care of a pile of mending in a short time. If you do not sew, you can take everything to a seamstress, or better yet, learn to sew! The cost of a seamstress will be less than the replacement cost of most clothing. And if you are willing to try your hand at some simple sewing so you can mend things yourself, you will save even more.

"Sewing? Yikes!" You may be a little out of your comfort zone when we bring up the subject of sewing. We have heard every excuse for not trying this craft. Some say that they tried it once and failed. Others claim an inability to do anything creative or crafty with their hands. You may be intimidated by the whole idea of it, too scared or too timid to jump in and try it.

We want to dispel all your fears and encourage you to give sewing a chance. You may find a new hobby. At least, you will be pleased with yourself for saving a lot of money. Remember that one of our principles is to be a do-it-yourselfer. You may have to practice some patience and perseverance until you have the basics down. But we are sure you can learn to mend, if not make, your family's clothing.

Jo and Gwen have both made just about every mistake possible in their sewing efforts. Only a constant lack of funds kept them persevering. Jo has sewn on sleeves inside out and back-wards. Gwen's hems have been uneven. Sometimes their fab-ric choices have been inappropriate. As a young newlywed, Jo cut through the telephone cord while cutting out a dress on the living room floor.

Eventually, we learned how to sew a straight seam, follow instructions, and come up with some very nice-looking gar-ments. In fact, Jo's daughter is quite proud of the pretty dresses Jo makes for her. Gwen's kids are long grown up, and much of her sewing now is curtains, bed coverings, little gift items, and of course mending, but she used to sew for them.

Even if you never construct a dress from scratch, learning to do some simple sewing so that you can do a good job of mend-ing can save you a lot of money. Think for a moment about cloth-ing you may have in your closets that you cannot wear due to split seams or missing buttons. Think some more about what it would take to make them wearable again by mending. You will be surprised how easy these little fix-it jobs can be!

Most mending is pretty easy to do and requires just a few spe-cial tools that you can find at a fabric store. Hems can be sewn by hand or fixed with fusible hemming tape. Patches can be ironed on. Sew buttons on by hand. For these simple mending projects you will need a packet of needles, thread, straight pins in a pincushion, a sewing gauge, tape measure, sewing scissors, fusible hemming tape, thread, and an iron.

Other mending projects require a sewing machine. Seam repairs are best done on a machine, and some patches will stay on better if machine sewn after they have been ironed on. If a hem needs a ravel-proof edge, a machine will be needed. When you use a sewing machine, you will also need several bobbins to hold various colors of thread, a variety of needles for different fabrics, and a seam ripper.

Finding a reliable sewing machine that you enjoy using can be tricky. Jo has done just about every kind of sewing and mending you can imagine on her mother's fifty-five-year-old Singer sewing machine. It has been a hardworking, faithful machine all those years. In spite of its limitations, Jo made her own wedding dress, sewed complete wardrobes for herself and her children, made curtains, fashioned slipcovers, and kept her family's wardrobes in good repair using that old Singer. She has never found a machine she enjoys more.

Gwen has been sewing since she was ten years old. She learned to sew on a little featherweight (eleven-pound) Singer that she has just recently inherited from her mom. The first investment she made after high school when she was working was a Pfaff sewing machine. It was high tech in those days. It's not so high tech now, but it does what she needs done and still sews like a dream. On that machine she made all of her little girl's dresses, tailored her own suits and coats, made almost all of the window coverings she has ever needed, and even made slipcovers (a wrestling job for an octopus).

A sewing machine can be a major investment, so we need to be careful in selecting one. Begin by asking people who sew a lot what they would recommend. Always try sewing on a machine before you buy it. Decide how many fancy stitches you really need and which options, bells, and whistles you can live without. You will want a machine that at least does a zigzag stitch and buttonholes and has a good track record for staying out of the repair shop. In fact, you may want to contact a repair shop to get their advice on a good, reliable sewing machine.

Machines can be found at the usual shoestring places. Ask why the machine is being sold. Bring thread and fabric so that you can try sewing with it. Do not buy a machine that has no instruction booklet; you'll need it as time goes on. Don't buy a machine that isn't working, thinking you'll get it fixed. You have no idea how much that would cost. If you don't like the way it sews, don't buy it. It is frustrating to use a machine that continually needs adjustments and repairs. That takes all the joy out of sewing. One of the most common problems machines have is with the tension. Proper tension affects how good and secure the stitches are. Machines require regular cleanings and tune-ups to keep them in proper working order.

We know several women who own machines but do not use them because the machines don't sew right or are in need of repair. That featherweight sewing machine Gwen inherited is probably close to sixty-five years old. She had it conditioned and serviced and it still runs like a dream. So if you have a machine that's not working, either get it repaired or trade it for one that is more reliable.

Mending 101

Whether you have a little experience with sewing or none at all, we suggest you begin your new efforts at sewing and mending with something easy. Unless you are an accomplished seamstress, have lots of time, and are willing to tackle very hard tasks, we suggest you save the tricky fix-ups for later when you have more experience. Right now you can hire someone to do them. Challenging projects would include relining a garment, major refitting, tailoring, and replacing zippers in men's slacks. However, most of the common, everyday mending tasks are straight sewing that is easily done. We will walk you through the most common ones. Let's begin with buttons.

Buttons

Buttons fall off even the best of garments. Some clothing comes with extra buttons unobtrusively sewn to the facing near the hem or to an inside seam or provided in a little packet attached to the tag. Look for them before you shop for replacement buttons. You may be fortunate and still have the button that came off. When a button comes loose and starts to hang by its threads, no matter where you are or what you are doing, pull it off and put it in your pocket. Better to go for a short time with no button than to have to buy a complete set of replacement buttons.

What if you do not have any matching buttons? Jo once lost a pearly button on a dress blouse. She used a button from the bottom of the blouse, the part that is always tucked in, to replace the missing button. She then found a button the right size and color from her collection of old buttons for the bottom of the blouse. Although the button did not match, no one ever saw it because it was tucked in. In fact, because Jo used a flat button instead of the rounded button that was there before, she eliminated the tiny bulge that button had previously created under her skirt on her tummy.

It takes a while to accumulate a button collection. You can buy bags of buttons pretty cheaply at fabric stores and even find them at garage sales and thrift stores on occasion. Or you can slowly and methodically collect them as we have done.

Recently Jo and her daughter sat down with a pile of clothing that was about to be discarded. With seam rippers and scissors they removed all the buttons and put them in Jo's button tin. Our button collections also grow whenever buttons are left over from craft and sewing projects. Over the years, our collections have grown so much that we rarely need to buy new buttons for replacements.

Gwen's mother used to keep her extra buttons in tin Lipton tea canisters. That tells you how long she had been collecting buttons. Who of us even knew tea came in tin canisters? When Gwen and her brothers cleaned out her parents' house, Gwen laid claim to those tins of buttons. The only problem is that now she is not sure which buttons are valuable antiques and which are everyday, run-of-the-mill buttons she can use.

Perhaps you have not been doing craft and sewing projects long enough to have accumulated a lot of buttons. If you are starting from scratch and there are no extra buttons sewn into the garment or hidden places in the garment to borrow from, it is time to shop. Take the whole garment with you to the fabric store or remove one button and just take that. You will be impressed with the wide selection of buttons, usually arranged according to categories and colors. Matching your button sounds simple, but it may not be. Watch carefully to get the best match in color and size.

What if you cannot find matching buttons? Then you have to find buttons that will work for the garment and replace all of them. Be sure to match the size perfectly. Color and style are up to you. This may be the time to update or give a new look to a garment by changing the buttons on it, as Gwen did with her navy blue jacket. If you do not feel confident in changing the look, pick something as close to the existing buttons as possible.

Sewing on buttons is an easy procedure that only requires needle and thread. Some sewing machines have the capability of sewing on buttons by using a zigzag stitch the width of the button holes and by dropping the feed dog (the little teeth on the sewing machine that pull the fabric through) so that the button and garment will not move. Follow the instructions that came with your sewing machine. Sometimes it is less trouble to sew by hand, especially for just one button.

There are two basic kinds of buttons: buttons with holes and buttons with shanks. Most shirts have buttons with holes. They are easy to sew on. Again, you will need some basic sewing tools: a needle, thread the same color that was used to sew on the button in the first place (look at the other buttons if the thread is gone), scissors, a toothpick, and the button.

You should be able to figure out where the missing button goes. There may be little holes left by the thread, the thread itself may remain, or there may be an indentation from the button. If none of these clues exist, button the garment and put a pin in the button's position under the buttonhole. Make sure the pin is in line with the other buttons.

Sewing On Buttons with Holes

1. Cut about twenty-four inches of thread. Thread the needle. Bring the ends of the thread together and knot them together. Tip: This job will go much quicker if you use four or even six strands of thread in your needle, because you will have to go in and out of the holes fewer times if you use multiple threads. Use a needle with an eye that will accommodate the thickness of more than one thread.

2. On the outside of the fabric, push the needle in and out to make a tiny (⅛-inch) stitch where the center of the button will be. Pull the needle until the knot stops the thread. The thread, needle, and knot should be on the right side of the fabric. When you are finished, the button will hide the knot.

3. Insert the needle through one of the holes in the button, going up through the bottom of the button and coming out the top. If the other buttons on the garment have a thread shank, you will want to create one on this button, as well. To do that put a toothpick on top of the button so that you will sew over it. This will create enough extra thread to make a shank.

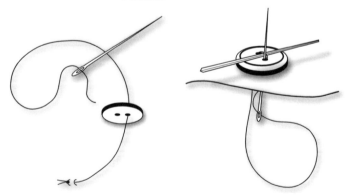

4. With the thumb of your nonsewing hand, hold the button exactly where you want it on the garment. Push the needle through another hole in the button, going from the top of the button down through the button and fabric and coming out on the inside of the garment.

5. Continue sewing up and down through the button as before, about three times. If your button has four holes, make two rows of parallel stitches through the holes. Don't crisscross threads to make an X.

6. If you are making a shank, make a final pass down through a hole in the button, but not through the fabric. Remove the toothpick. You will find that the button has a little space between it and the fabric when pulled firmly up. Encircle the shank of thread between the button and the fabric with the remaining thread about five times, then push the needle and thread to the inside of the fabric.

7. To make the thread and button secure, you will need to knot the thread. Make sure your needle and thread are on the wrong side of the fabric. Make a tiny stitch in the middle of the stitches you made when you were sewing on the button, pulling the thread until there is a small loop left. Put the needle through that loop and pull until taut. Repeat this step one more time to make sure you have a good knot. Clip the thread and you are done!

Sewing On Shank Buttons

Shank buttons are sewn on much the same way as buttons with holes.

1. Begin as before, following steps 1 and 2 on previous page, then pulling the needle and thread through the hole in the shank.

2. With your thumb, hold the button so its top is resting on the fabric next to its position. Push the needle back down through the fabric close to where the needle last came out. Repeat to sew three loops through the hole in the shank.

3. Push the needle up through from the wrong side of the fabric to the right side, but do not go through the shank. Instead, wrap the thread around the thread shank you made with the previous stitches, then push the needle through to the wrong side of the fabric and knot as described above.

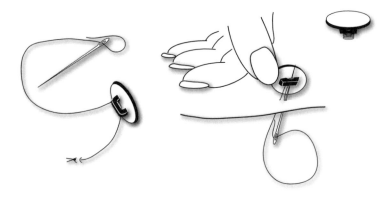

Wow! That was easy! Now you can wear that blouse without embarrassment. Fixing that button didn't take long once you got everything together. Speaking of which, you might want to get organized so it is not such a big deal every time you need to sew on a button. Gather all your sewing tools in one place such as a basket or drawer. Make it a place easily accessible to minimize any hassle. The sewing basket may include needles, pins, pincushion, threads in assorted basic colors, a needle threader, tape measure, small ruler or sewing gauge, a button collection, and scissors. Those scissors are meant only for sewing, by the way. If they are used for all kinds of household projects, you may have to hunt for them every time you want to use them. Cutting paper with your sewing scissors will dull them. Have a separate place for other scissors and office supplies.

Mending a Split Seam

Everyone experiences a split seam now and then. This happens when the threads in the seam have worn out or have been stressed beyond their strength, but the fabric is still in good shape. This problem often occurs in the crotch of pants. Let's use that situation to lead you through the simple steps to mending a split seam.

Before you begin, you will need to get thread that is the same color as the thread used in making the pants or that is the same color as the garment. This mending can be done by hand but you will end up with a stronger seam if you use a machine. Set the stitch size to between twelve and fourteen stitches per inch. Be sure the needle on the machine is appropriate for the fabric you will be using. Needle packages have guidelines printed on them to help you with that decision. You will also need other basic sewing tools such as pins and scissors, and if you are like us and require more than one try to get it right, you will also need a seam ripper.

Turn the pants inside out. If the garment is lined, you must get between the lining and the fabric to do the repair. That can mean taking out the stitches that hold the lining to the garment, then resewing them when you are done mending. Once you have the pants inside out, you may discover that both the seams that meet in the crotch have come apart. You will need to sew the leg seams first and then the crotch seam in jeans; do the reverse in fleece warm-up pants. Study the garment you are mending to figure out what should be done first. Begin by carefully pinning the first seam where you need to sew. Keep the edges of the fabric even. You should be able to see where the stitches of the worn-out seam had been. Look for tiny holes left by the stitches or a slight fold where the seam folded open.

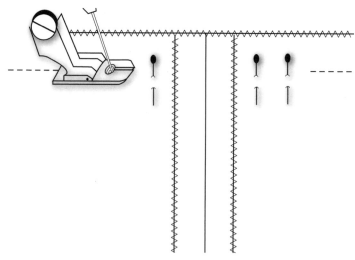

Place the pants under the sewing foot of your machine so that your new stitching will begin before the split in the seam. Back tack (sew forward and backward with the machine) a few stitches, then carefully sew on the old seam line. Sew past the split if it is in the middle of a seam or to the end of the material if possible. As you sew, remove each pin as you come to it. Do not sew over the pins if you can help it because you will dull your sewing machine needle, ruin your pin, and possibly even sew the seam a tiny bit off track. Back tack again at the end of the mending. Trim all loose threads as close to the pants as you can.

Turn the pants right side out and see how your sewing looks. You should see no obvious signs that the pants have been mended. Otherwise you may need to painstakingly remove your stitches and try again. Better to keep trying till you get it right than to have a pair of pants you are afraid to be seen in from behind.

Press the completed seam open, and while you are at it, press the entire pair of pants so they are ready to wear. You have saved time and a bundle of money because you don't have to go shopping for another pair.

Shortening Skirts

Jo's daughter Anna recently acquired a skirt that was too long for her. To shorten it, Jo could have just folded up the hem and sewn it in place with the sewing machine. But that would have looked so bad. With just a little extra effort, Jo hemmed the skirt the right way and got professional-looking results. It was worth the extra time to do it right.

Some skirts are almost impossible to shorten with any success. This includes skirts with pleats permanently creased or sewn in; the pleats near the new hem will never look right. Skirts cut on the bias (cut diagonal to the warp and woof—threads that go up and down and those that go across) can be very tricky and should be reserved for more experienced sewers. Some fabrics are extremely difficult to work with. Anything silky, gauzy, or stretchy falls into that category. If you are doubtful, take it to an expert who is used to working with these kinds of fabrics and can do it well. It might be worth the expense to prevent frazzled nerves. Jo once offered to shorten a dress for a friend before she saw what it was like. She ended up in tears trying to hem the fabric that not only was cut on the bias but was stretchy and gauzy as well. "Never again!" she said.

Hopefully these warnings haven't scared you off. Most skirts are easily shortened and require little skill. We will teach you two ways to shorten a skirt. The first way is to simply trim off the hem and sew in a new hem. But another way that is especially good for a growing girl's clothes is to sew in tucks near the hem on the outside of the skirt, creating a decorative element. As the child grows, the tucks can be taken out to make the skirt longer. This method was often used when making dresses for young ladies in the earlier part of the century.

We will begin with the first method. You will need a needle, matching thread, scissors, a hem gauge or ruler, pins, yardstick, and a sewing machine. Some people use tailor's chalk to mark the new hem length, but pins work just fine. To hem a skirt by cutting off the excess material:

1. Begin by deciding what kind of hem to put in the skirt. The easiest answer to that question is found in the skirt itself. You will want to duplicate the original hem and edge finishing as closely as possible. How deep was the first hem? Hems on a skirt or dress should never be more than $2\frac{1}{2}$ inches deep. Was any fabric folded under to keep the edges from unraveling? Were the edges finished with a zigzag type of stitch?

2. The next step is to remove the old hem's stitching and press out the crease in the fabric. Pressing will make the fabric easier to work with and you will be able to achieve a more even hem. Be very careful when you wield a seam ripper or scissors; you do not want to accidentally snip the fabric.

3. Next, have the person who will be wearing the skirt put it on. We will refer to her as our "model." She should look in a full-length mirror with you to decide on the desired new length. Pin the skirt up to see if it is the right length. Then remove all but one of the pins and have the model stand on a sturdy, level stool.

4. Using a yardstick, measure from the floor to where the new hem length is pinned on the skirt. Write down that measurement so you do not forget it. Remove that last pin.

5. Use the yardstick to measure all the way around the skirt, pinning it or using tailor's chalk to mark the same measurement all the way around. Be sure to keep the yardstick straight to ensure accurate measuring. You can either

walk around the model as you measure or have her turn. The model can now carefully (remember the pins!) remove the skirt.

6. Figure out how deep the hem needs to be and add ¼ inch to your measurement if you will be turning the edge of the fabric under to create a ravel-free edge. Measure and mark that distance down from the pins all the way around the skirt. The higher marking (the pins you put in while the model had the skirt on) is the length the skirt will be; the lower marking is where you must cut the skirt to have enough fabric left to turn under and still achieve the desired length. Cut off the excess fabric at the lower marking.

7. Now you have to finish the fabric edges to make sure they do not unravel. You do not want threads hanging down looking tacky, tickling your legs, and telling all the world that your skirt is unraveling. For the kind of hem edging that is turned under ¼ inch, press the ¼-inch fabric allowance under to make it easier to sew. Use a ruler or hem sewing guide to make sure you are turning under a consistent width. Then run a line of stitching with the sewing machine to make sure that ¼-inch edging stays in place. Use thread that matches the color of the garment.

If your choice of edging is zigzag, you will need a sewing machine that can do a zigzag stitch. Practice on the fabric you cut off earlier to get an idea of how to do it and how the fabric will respond to zigzagging. Some fabric will stretch when being zigzagged. Experiment with different widths and lengths of stitches and figure out exactly how close to the edge of the fabric you will stitch to get the best results. When you are happy with your results, do the edging of the hem.

8. Now for the real hem. You are almost there. It takes as long to read about shortening a hem as it takes to do it—

well, almost! Fold the hem on the hemline you marked when the model stood on the stool. Press the new hem in place and pin it every two inches to hold it securely. Place the pins ½ inch from the finished edge of the hem. If there seems to be too much fabric when you start pinning the hem up, do not make little tucks and folds in the hem. That will look bulky and unprofessional from the front side. To eliminate the problem, run a gathering stitch around the edge of the hem. This is usually the largest stitch your sewing machine can make. Then when you find too much fullness in part of the hem while pinning, you can just pull up the thread in the gathering stitches to make soft gathers. Sometimes pulling up the thread tightens the fabric just enough to eliminate any fullness without making any gathers. Once you are done pinning, sew the hem in place using the best type of stitch for the garment. (Two methods of sewing in hems are given below.)

The two basic types of hems used by home sewers are machine-made topstitch and the blind stitch. You'll have to decide which you prefer, but using what was done on the old hem is a good guideline.

Machine-Made Topstitch

The machine-made topstitch is easily done using the sewing machine. Denim and other crisp fabrics look good with machine-made topstitched hems. Knits will curl and stretch if you sew them too close to the edge with a machine.

The trick to making a nice looking machine-made topstitch is to sew a straight line, especially since it will be visible from the outside of the skirt. A straight line is easily achieved when making a very narrow, ¼-inch hem by keeping the side of the sewing foot on the edge of the hem. Jo's mother taught her to put tape on the sewing machine parallel to the long edge of the sewing foot to use as a guide. It works nicely.

Begin and end machine sewing on the underside of the skirt at the center back seam. Use about eight stitches per inch, or stitches about ⅛ inch long. Back tack a few stitches at the end to secure the stitching. Press the skirt again and wear with pride.

Blind Stitch

The blind stitch is usually done by hand, although your machine may have the capability. Your machine's instruction book can help you there. For the handmade hem stitch, you just need to learn one simple stitch. You will be very good at it by the time you are done with one skirt. To hem with a blind stitch:

1. Cut about twenty-four inches of thread that matches the skirt. Thread a needle. Leave one end of the thread short—about six inches through the needle—and knot the end of the long piece. If your thread is too long, it will get tangled and knotted. You do not need that extra frustration.

2. Beginning at the center back seam, turn back a bit of the hem and make a tiny stitch near the edge.

3. Fold the hem back to the pins marking the desired length. Make tiny stitches, picking up only a couple threads from the skirt; then pick up a couple threads from the hem, about ¼ inch from the edge. Continue making stitches ¼ inch apart, pulling the thread just taut enough to make a sturdy hem, but not tight enough to make the skirt pucker. The hem stitching should be almost invisible from the outside side of the skirt.

4. When you've hemmed all the way around the skirt, securely knot the thread by making a tiny stitch at the edge of the hem and pulling the thread only until a small loop is left. Put the needle through the loop and pull the

thread taut. Repeat to make a double knot. Clip the thread near the knot.

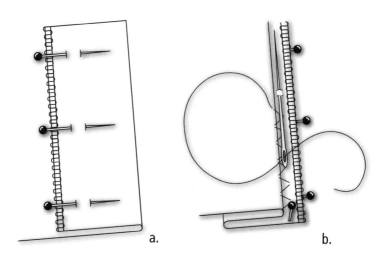

a.   b.

5. Remove all the pins, press the skirt, and wear it with pride!

Instead of sewing a hem, some claim it is quicker to iron it in place using fusible webbing. This product is sold in fabric stores. To use it, carefully follow the instructions that come with it. It may not take hard wear or rough washing and does not work on every type of fabric, so read the package thoroughly to see if this kind of hem is appropriate for your skirt.

Sewing Tucks into Skirts

In the good old days that ended just a few decades ago, little girls' dresses and skirts were frequently made with rows of tucks above the hems. Many yards of fabric were required to make a dress, so most little girls did not own very many dresses. These dresses were a lot of trouble to sew by hand and the fabric was expensive. So tucks that could be removed to lengthen the dress or skirt as the young girl grew were sewn in when the garment was constructed. Sewing in tucks saved the family a great deal of time and money because when a girl got taller, all they had to do was let out the tucks.

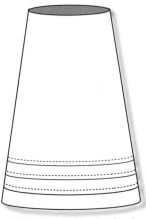

Even today you will sometimes find rows of tucks sewn onto fancy party dresses. They are there as decorative details only, as most people are not aware of their original usage. It does not take a lot of trouble to make these tucks in an existing dress to shorten it or to add them when you are sewing a new dress for your daughter or when fixing up a thrifty find.

The tucks are usually about one inch deep, which shortens the skirt by two inches. You can make them thinner or thicker, and you can sew in as many as you like. Experiment using pins to temporarily secure the tucks to see how many you need or want. If you are working with a dress rather than just a skirt, you might want to add matching tucks to the sleeves not only to use for lengthening later but also to carry the same detail throughout the garment. Use a ruler or sewing gauge to make sure you make the tucks even along the bottom of the skirt. Use fairly large stitches (about six to eight per inch) to make them easier to remove in the future. The tucks look best when placed several inches above the hem.

Hemming Slacks

Most pants and slacks can be hemmed using the same steps described for making straight hems in skirts. Denim jeans may be too thick for your machine to stitch through all the layers required to hem them. If the pant legs are tapered, a bunchy looking hem may result when a new hem is sewn in place because the width of the hemmed edge is less than the width a couple inches higher where the hem is attached.

157

You can follow our hemming instructions to hem just about anything. Follow this guide for hem depths:

- $\frac{5}{8}$ to $1\frac{1}{4}$ inch for T-shirt sleeves
- $1\frac{1}{4}$ to $1\frac{1}{2}$ inch for shorts and slacks
- $1\frac{1}{2}$ to 2 inches for jackets
- 2 to 3 inches for straight skirts and coats

PATCHES

Little children spend a lot of time playing on their knees. As a result, kids get holes in the knees of their pants before they grow out of them. Usually all but the knees of the pants are still in good condition. Some children's pants are made with extra thickness sewn into the knees. This really helps. Sometimes, however, Junior, pushing his truck all over his world, will wear out even the sturdiest pair of pants. It's time for patches. Patches can double the life of your child's play clothes and therefore save you money. If you are covering a tear in a garment, first sew the tear so that it will not grow under the "fix."

Iron-On Patches

The easiest type of patch to use is an iron-on patch. These come in packages at fabric stores. Heavyweight patches are generally available in light blue denim, dark blue denim, brown, green, gray, and tan. Patches for lighter weight clothing are available in a variety of colors. Patching material can also be purchased in large sheets or in patch sizes of five-by-five or two-by-three inches. You can cut one large patch into two small ones. Just be sure the patch completely covers the worn area and a little bit of unworn area around it. Follow the instructions given on the package for applying the patches. All you will need is an iron. Wash the pants first to remove any dirt that might prevent a strong bond.

158

You will also find tiny decorative iron-on patches at the fabric store. They come in various sports themes, flowers, stars, hearts, and other designs. By adding one over a hole on the knee of the pants and a matching one to the pocket of a shirt, you have made your patching look like part of the original design. These little patches are usually not more than an inch or two in width, so they are only good for hiding small holes in garments. They can be easily ironed on to create a bit of whimsy on an otherwise dull pair of jeans or warm-up pants.

A visit to the notions section of a fabric store reveals many other options for mending with iron-on materials. You will find a wide selection of fusible tapes and also a spray-on adhesive that enables you to create your own iron-on patch. Spend some time studying the products to see what will meet your needs. New products are constantly being developed.

Iron-on patches will last longer if you use your machine to sew around the edges of the patch, or you can whipstitch the edges in place by hand.

How to Sew a Whipstitch:

1. Thread a needle with about twenty-four inches of thread that matches the garment. Bring both ends of the thread together and knot. You will be sewing with a double thread.

2. From the inside of the garment, push the threaded needle up through the fabric along the outside edge of the patch—not putting the needle into the patch but just adjacent to it.

3. Stab the needle into the patch about $\frac{1}{8}$ inch further long the edge and $\frac{1}{8}$ inch into the edge of the patch. Pull the needle down through the fabric, coming out on the inside.

4. Push the needle back up through the garment, $\frac{1}{8}$ inch farther along the edge of the patch, close to its edge.

Continue sewing down through the patch and up through the garment near the edge of the patch. Completely finish the edge of the patch this way, then knot the thread on the underside of the garment as described in the hemming section.

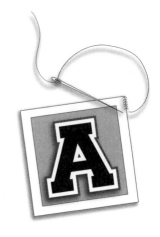

Sewn-on Patches

An alternative and less expensive way to patch pants is to use a sturdy fabric and your sewing machine. When our kids were young and wearing out the knees of their jeans at an alarming rate, we kept worn-out jeans and used the less-worn parts of the denim to make patches. Try to use the same kind of fabric (denim, fleece, sailcloth, and so forth) to make a patch. Your patches can be of contrasting colors. Be creative. The patch will need to have finished edges so it will not unravel. Either carefully make a $1/4$-inch hem all the way around the edge or zigzag the edge. Be sure the patch is large enough to cover the hole plus some unworn fabric around it. In other words, although the hole in your son's jeans may be only one inch wide, the pale areas around it showing wear need to be covered also. Sewing a new patch where the fabric is worn will not create a strong mend. You will have to sew the patch onto the darker area that looks unworn, like the rest of the pants.

To patch pants, use a seam ripper or scissors to remove the inner leg seam. Opening the leg will give you access to one layer of fabric, making it easier to work with. After you have opened a pant leg, lay it flat on a hard surface. Pin the patch in place, placing the pins an inch apart, perpendicular to the edge. Some seamstresses prefer to use fusible webbing to hold the patch in place so that it will not slip when being sewn down. Hold up the pants to check the placement of the patch and to make sure it is straight.

Unless you have used fusible webbing to hold the patch in place, you may want to ensure correct positioning by either hand basting the patch or using a large machine stitch to baste it in place. (Basting stitches are large stitches meant only to hold things in place while they are being permanently sewn down.) Again, check your work before proceeding. Patches tend to slip, turn, and do funny things unless they are very well secured before the final sewing. When you are sure of the placement and that the patch will not shift around and sabotage your efforts, you are ready to sew. With thread that matches either the pants or the patch, use a smallish stitch, about ten to twelve stitches per inch, very close to the edge of the patch. You may prefer to use a zigzag stitch with stitches close together to make it look like an appliqué.

Again, inspect your work. If you are pleased with the results, sew the inner leg seam, and you are done. While you have all the supplies out, you may want to patch both knees even though only one has holes. Our experience tells us that the other knee will soon be worn through as well. Two patches look as if the pants were designed that way!

By now you may be thinking that we are overcautious, making you check and double-check to make sure the patch doesn't shift while it is being sewn on. This is the voice of experience speaking. We have learned over the years that checking and rechecking prevents disasters. It is so depressing to discover that the patch is crooked or that it hides bunched fabric beneath it. To have to remove the inner leg seam again (while wiping away tears and sniffling), then remove the tiny stitches holding the patch (exercising self-control as naughty words come to the tip of our tongue), and then begin all over again is such a waste of time and *so* frustrating. Do it right, carefully, and cautiously the first time, and you will save yourself much grief—and time.

Simple Sewing

Did you take a sewing or home economics class sometime in your distant past? Dig out the dusty textbook if you still have it. It's time to polish your rusty sewing skills!

Did you just say to yourself that you never, ever, in your whole life learned the first thing about sewing? There is still hope for you. Find someone who sews and trade lessons for baby-sitting or some other skill. Fabric stores and sewing machine stores offer classes. Your community college or city recreation department may offer classes as well. Now, no more excuses!

Once you get the hang of sewing—and you will if you keep at it—you will be amazed how handy it is and how much money you can save. We do not recommend sewing every garment your family wears, although some people find that doable, but we do suggest you learn not only to mend but also to sew some simple garments. Many costumes required for school plays and fun dress-up clothing fall into the "easy to sew" category. You will find sewing one of the handiest skills you ever learned. Be sure to pass this skill on to your children so they can benefit all their lives as well.

At this point we wish we could provide you with a complete textbook, a selection of patterns for the beginning seamstress, and a teaching video. Unfortunately, we can't give you more extensive instructions here. Better and more experienced seamstresses than we are have produced books and videos. Find them at your local library and use them.

Our friend Sally Frazzle has decided to revive her long-lost sewing lessons from junior high school and make a simple blouse to go with that lonely skirt in her closet that she has never worn because it matches nothing. We are going to spy on her to pick up some pointers.

Sally's Adventure in Sewing

Although it is a wet, chilly, gloomy Saturday, Sally wakes up with hope. Today she is going to make a blouse. Or at least get started. Last weekend everyone seemed to have a reason to blow the budget, so some corners have to be cut and some compromises have to be made. Bruce is going to earn money to buy his own basketball shoes. Ted has decided to save for a couple of shirts and a new suit. Spacy is learning to be content and is now responsible for doing the family laundry so she cannot complain about her favorite things not being clean. And Sally has decided to begin to fill in some wardrobe needs by sewing a blouse. They all agreed that they would not spend money they do not have.

Sally did her homework at the mall where she visited the Dillard's and JCPenney department stores. She studied a few fashion magazines at the library and noted what style of blouse works well with her skirt. It is a fairly enduring, classic design that will look stylish for a few years. She doesn't want to go to all the trouble of sewing a blouse and then only be able to wear it for one season. She has written in a little notebook next to a sketch of the blouse that her blouse will be made of a nice light-weight cotton fabric in a cheerful stripe that coordinates with the skirt.

At home she cleaned the sewing machine, gathered her sewing supplies, and cleared her Saturday schedule. She even unearthed her old sewing notebook from home economics class. After reviewing a few pages, she is sure she can still do this.

At the fabric store, with her skirt in a shopping bag and her notebook tucked into the outer pocket of her purse, Sally begins to peruse the pattern catalogs. She finds just what she wants in two different catalogs but decides to buy a pattern that also includes some other blouses she might want to make in the future. The blouse is very simple, without difficult tucks, collars, complicated lines, or too many buttons. She writes down the number of the pattern in the notebook, then finds the pattern in the serve-yourself pattern drawers. Each pattern envelope contains several sizes so Sally picks out the pattern she thinks will fit. Coincidentally, her chosen brand of patterns are all ninety-nine cents this weekend. This particular store usually sells all its patterns 50 percent off, which really helps as patterns have become very expensive in the past few years.

Sally now chooses her fabric. The store contains a rainbow of rows and rows of beautiful choices. Sally must remember what she is looking for and not be tempted or distracted by the many other fabrics. She wanders around until she finds just what she needs. She chooses a lightweight cotton with just enough polyester to keep the fabric from wrinkling too much. The fabric matches her skirt perfectly. As she winds her way through rows of fabrics toward the cutting table, she studies the back of the pattern envelope to decide how much fabric she will need. The amount varies according to sizes. Now there is a problem. If she remembers correctly, the size of a blouse you buy at a department store is not the same as the pattern size you need. Back to the pattern books. In the back of the catalog where she found her pattern, she finds a list of measurements for each size. Sally suddenly realizes that she has no clue what her measurements are. And she has not yet learned to carry a retractable tape measure in her purse. She recalls seeing some colorful little tape measures in a basket by the cash register near the front of the store, so she gets one and takes it to a back corner of the store, behind the tall bolts of upholstery fabric, to surreptitiously measure herself.

After recovering from the shock of the numbers ("I am going to start dieting and exercising today," she says to herself), Sally checks the pattern catalog again to figure out her size. Her measurements do not exactly match any particular size so she picks the size that fits her bust measurement since she will be making a blouse.

Back to the cutting table Sally confidently goes. She asks the nice employee to cut the required amount of fabric from the bolt. The thoughtful lady then asks her if she needs anything else such as thread or buttons. Sally is grateful for this sales pitch because she does indeed require both thread and a couple of buttons. The back of the pattern envelope usually lists any notions that are needed to construct each garment. In Sally's case, the list includes thread and two $\frac{1}{2}$-inch buttons.

At the checkout counter Sally returns the tape measure to the basket, then thinks again. This little gadget could come in handy, and it is only two dollars. She decides to buy it. As the cashier rings up the total, Sally is pleased to note that it is much less than the blouse would have cost at a department store.

At home she spreads the fabric on her clean kitchen table. Sally adjusts the fabric so the edges are even and it is lying flat and straight. The illustration for laying out the pattern pieces (included with the pattern) for the blouse is pretty easy to follow. The pattern pieces are full of wrinkles and folds that make it hard to lay them out accurately, so Sally presses them flat with a warm iron. She pins them on the fabric, making sure they are placed straight with the grain of fabric and that the center front is on the fold, not on a disconnected edge of the fabric. (If the pattern were placed on an edge other than the fold, you would end up with two pieces for the front of the blouse rather than just one.) Not wanting to ruin everything, she double-checks to make sure she has used pattern pieces for the style she wants in the size she needs and that all the pieces are there. Everything seems to be correct. Taking a deep breath, Sally begins to cut the fabric around the pattern pieces. She is very meticulous about cutting right on the cutting lines. Before removing the pins, she uses tracing paper to mark where the darts and buttons will go. All those warnings and lessons from her home economics teacher are coming back to her. Now that she is spending *her* hard-earned money and not her parents', she is motivated to do the job right.

After a quick lunch, Sally feels ready to begin sewing. She replaces the needle in her machine with the type appropriate for her fabric and puts the thread she bought in the machine, then makes a seam in a scrap of fabric to ensure the tension and stitch size are okay. It seems to be all systems go, so Sally sews her first seams with a loose basting stitch. The directions that come with the pattern take some getting used to. Sally has to go back to the first page of the instructions to see what all the symbols mean and how to do a few things like finish the seams.

After the side and shoulder seams are basted with big stitches, Sally tries on the blouse to see if it will fit as it is or will need some slight altering. She has her daughter pin the back of the blouse to mimic how it will close when the buttons are in place. This will give her a true picture of the fit. Sally and Spacy agree that the blouse looks like a perfect fit. Now Sally is ready to sew the seams with smaller stitches and then finish each raw edge with a zigzag stitch.

As Sally sews, she follows the pattern instructions and recalls her home economics teacher's constant mantra: "Press! Press! Press as you go!" This takes a little longer, but Sally knows that the finished garment will look much better if she presses each seam open as she progresses.

A couple of hours later, after being more careful and meticulous than she has ever been in her life, Sally has a beautiful new blouse that fits her. It is amazingly similar to the blouse she wanted at Dillard's.

On a shoestring high, she fixes her family a healthy meal instead of buying take-out pizza, thereby saving even more money this weekend. They may even stay within their budget this month! Sally thinks she may even be successful at restyling some of her family's still good but outdated clothing!

SHOESTRING TIPS

1. Find a tin or other storage container and begin your own button collection.

2. Get your sewing machine fixed, tuned up, and cleaned.

3. Learn how to sew.

4. Practice sewing straight seams with scraps of fabric.

5. Spend an hour in a fabric store to see the many tools available to help you in mending and sewing.

6. Put together a sewing kit. You may find them already assembled for you at fabric stores, especially during the Christmas season. Could someone give you one as a gift?

7. Check out the sewing how-to books at the library. They can give you a lot more detailed advice and help than we have given in this book.

8. While you are at the library, peruse some fashion magazines for new ideas.

9. Search fabric stores for mending aids. You will find all kinds of fusible materials, fabric glue, replacement buttons and buckles for overalls, an automatic button-fastener called the Buttoneer, fix-it strips for emergency temporary mends, replacement hooks and straps for bras, bra extenders for the back of bras, and much more.

NINE

RESTYLING WHAT
YOU HAVE

We hate to throw away a great piece of clothing. It goes against our shoestring grain! Our parents trained us to use, reuse, and reuse again anything with any possibilities. And so we have learned to restyle clothing. A beautiful wool jacket in a color we love is hard to get rid of!

Already you have seen how Gwen changed the buttons on a jacket to extend its life, and you can imagine how many times we have added or removed trim to update our kids' clothing. In this chapter we hope to inspire you to take another look at the clothing you would ordinarily get rid of.

In fact, with a little effort, your own closets can become one of the best sources for clothing your family on a shoestring budget. By restyling what you have, mending favorites that have been hanging idle for some time, shortening dresses and skirts to a more fashionable length, altering pants or jackets that are too snug or too loose, or replacing outdated buttons, you can have lots of clothes for the price of a little trim or some new buttons and your time. So let's plunge into that closet and see what we can do to give you and your family more clothing.

Restyling Your Outdated Clothing

You get to exercise a lot of creativity in restyling your clothing. Choose garments of good quality—ones that are too good to throw out but are just not quite right for the times. With a little creativity and Yankee ingenuity, you may be able to remove, change, or disguise the details that make it so "yesterday."

Jo recently took an outdated, black, fully lined, linen jacket with shoulders that were too broad to be in style any longer and remade it. She took an entire day to fuss, pin, pin again, and pin yet again, then sew, rip, and sew again. She removed, trimmed, and then replaced the shoulder pads. She narrowed the shoulders. Then she made the long sleeves short and the whole thigh-length jacket into a cropped-style short jacket. It was a lot of work, but without any outlay of cash she ended up with a very stylish, becoming jacket that looks great with her long white linen pleated skirt.

Some things are beyond hope for restyling. Things that are too worn are not good candidates. Fabrics that have become faded, pilled, thin, yellowed, or stretched out of shape are hopeless. If the fabric was cheap in the first place, there is nothing you can do to make it look like great quality. Your '70s polyester knit is not a candidate for a remodeling project. There is nothing you can do to make a '70s polyester knit up-to-date. But if we are working with a good wool gabardine, 100 percent cotton, linen, or a blend that may include polyester, the project may well be worth your time.

Maybe you should go through your discard pile again to see if you have some candidates for restyling that you previously planned to discard. Are there things in that pile that have small rips or stains? Don't throw them out yet. There may still be hope. We'll give you some ideas below.

Some styles from years ago have come back into style. Gwen wears a 1950s black, wool crew neck sweater that is right in style. So before you toss out or restyle all your relics, check at a good department store. You might just see something very similar to what's hanging in your closet. Then you won't have to restyle the garment.

Keep an open mind about how you can remake an outfit or separate garments. Maybe that little pants and shirt set with the big hole in the knee could have a new life as a shorts set. Will the shirt look good with jeans, overalls, or a jumper? Can a dress that is too short be made into a tunic? Perhaps the fabric in a hand-me-down can be used to make something else entirely. Full-skirted dresses have yards of material. Don't forget to recycle the zipper and buttons as well. Jo has even used old clothing to make dresses for her daughter's dolls. Both Gwen and Jo have slept under patchwork quilts that were made from the good parts of old clothing. One of Jo's friends collected old plaid garments until she had enough to make a patchwork full-length skirt for festive winter occasions.

HIDING PROBLEMS

You may have some clothing that needs to be restyled to hide a stain or tear. This can be done several ways. You can use a patch, as described earlier. Other alternatives include pockets, trim, buttons, and bows. Remember to sew the tear so that it will not grow under the "fix."

Pockets

Pockets can be added to almost any garment. If a stain or rip is close to where a pocket would normally be placed, you can add one to cover the problem. The trick is to make the garment look as if it has always had a pocket. To do this, you will have to use the same fabric you use for the new pocket somewhere else on the outfit. Use it as another pocket or as trim for a collar, cuff, or band. Carefully choose the fabric. Use the same type of fabric originally used for the garment if you can. Make sure the pocket or patch is the same weight, has been prewashed, and will require the same care in washing as the original garment. If a garment is faded from multiple washings, a new fabric patch will not look good. You might need to find a worn piece of fabric.

Let us use a little girl's church dress to see how this works. Let's say the dress is a pink flowered print with a white collar, puffed sleeves with white bands, a full skirt, and a white ribbon for a sash. There is a stain on the front skirt of the dress where red punch was spilled. Adding a pocket of the same white material that was used on the collar and sleeve bands can hide the stain. To further tie it in with the rest of the dress, pink rosettes can be attached to the top of the pocket, on each sleeve band, and on the collar. Now your problem stain has become a decorative addition to the dress.

A two-piece shorts outfit in a red, white, and blue print for a little boy may require a slightly different solution. It has a hole right in the middle of the shirt front where the little boy's tummy met a sharp object. This is not the right place for a pocket, but adding a band of red, white, or blue fabric would coordinate with the outfit and cover the hole. Make the band at least an inch wide. It only needs to be added to the front, so you may have to remove a few stitches from the side seams, tuck the ends of the bands in, sew the band on, and then sew the seam again. Then use the same fabric to add bands to the shorts about an inch or two from the hems. Perhaps you can also add a pocket of the same fabric to the front or back of the shorts.

Bands of fabric are not the only way to hide problems. Your fabric store has a wide selection of ribbons, flowers made of ribbons, patches, buttons, lace, ruffled lace, and trims of all kinds. Think about how you might use fabric paint too.

Another alternative for covering holes and stains is to add a design using the appliqué method. This is very similar to adding a patch as we discussed in chapter 8. Begin your appliqué by cutting a design out of another fabric. Make sure you prewash the new fabric first. Then attach it as you would a patch, using Wonder-Under bonding material or a similar adhesive product. Then zigzag stitch all around the edge. You can use this technique to add such things as your child's favorite cartoon or movie character to an existing garment.

In your fabric and craft store, you will also find designs that can be transferred to a shirt using an iron. While these designs may not cover a tear, they may cover a stain and also make the shirt look new and interesting. Stores have a wide range of designs to choose from, and these iron-ons require no sewing. An inexpensive man's T-shirt can be transformed into a pretty shirt for a girl or woman using these "transfers." If a shirt has a design that is worn or objectionable, you can hide the old design by ironing an updated design onto a large rectangle of fabric and then sewing the whole rectangle onto the shirt.

Collars and Cuffs

If you wear a garment that has a collar and cuffs for enough years, it will eventually fray. On women's and girls' shirts, you can take the collar off and replace it with a lace collar (you will find them ready-made at fabric stores). If you are adventurous, you could use a removed collar as a pattern for creating a new, updated collar. On men's shirts you can just take the collar off and restitch the band to make a collarless shirt. They've been popular for a number of years.

You can remove the collar and cuffs and replace them with a new collar and cuffs cut from a contrasting fabric, giving the garment an entirely new look. Dress up a basic long-sleeved dress by making lace bracelet cuffs (lace stitched onto elastic and worn like a bracelet).

Coats and shirts with worn knit cuffs can be revived by sewing on new cuffs available at fabric stores. The new cuffs come in a wide selection of colors and are ready to be put in place. This is a straightforward and simple sewing task. You simply remove the worn cuff and sew in the new one in its place.

Sleeves

Shortening Sleeves

The first and most obvious way to change a sleeve is to cut it off and make a long-sleeved shirt into a short-sleeved shirt. Just cut it off at the length you like plus an inch or so for a hem. If you really want to keep that cuff but the sleeve needs shortening, you can take out the stitching that holds the cuff in place, cut the sleeve to the length you want, slip the raw edge back into the cuff, and carefully restitch it with matching thread and the same stitch length.

You can also take tiny tucks in the lower sleeve to pull the cuff up to the right length. Do this by marking the sleeve carefully, using a washable marker, with several rows of parallel lines $\frac{1}{2}$ inch apart. Bring the lines together and pin or baste. Then stitch about $\frac{1}{2}$ inch from the edge to form a tuck. The result is very decorative and tailored looking, and the sleeve will be the right length.

It takes a little more work, but you can remove the sleeve at the shoulder seam, cut the excess fabric from the top, and resew it in place.

Lengthening Sleeves

Usually, if the sleeves are too short, the whole garment is too short and it is time to pass it on. However, some people have long arms and have a hard time finding sleeves long enough. Men's and boys' clothing tend to have longer sleeves, so some of our women friends shop those departments to find things that fit.

There are a couple of ways to make those things with inadequate sleeve lengths longer. The easiest way is to remove the cuffs, add an extension of a matching or contrasting fabric to the bottom of the sleeve, and make it a straight sleeve rather than a cuffed one.

Another trick is to add an inset into the sleeve below the elbow. Cut the sleeve about four inches above the cuff. Add an inset of lace or a contrasting fabric. Be sure to use that same lace or contrasting fabric elsewhere in the outfit so it will look like it was meant to be that way.

Trim

The trim on a garment can date it. Ask yourself if the garment needs any trim at all. If the answer is no, remove all trim, and be sure to pick out any little threads that may have remained. Steam the area where the trim was to remove all the indentations of the trim. Try sponging the area with white vinegar and then using a steam iron.

Children's clothing especially can be enhanced by the use of trim. If you have a lot of hand-me-downs, consider customizing them with trim. If you want to replace the trim, first go to a clothing store to see what kinds are in style. Then go to a fabric store prepared to be overwhelmed by the number of trims and decorative elements that are available. Let your imagination go wild. Here are some fixes that might start you thinking.

Add soutache or military braid to plain clothing for a decorative touch. Add decorative patches to cover stains and holes. Gwen has an outdoor jacket that she bought at a thrift shop for only a few dollars. It was a brand-new salesman's sample. A hole had been cut in the middle of the lower back to indicate it was a sample and to assure the manufacturer that the garment would not be sold at retail. Gwen really liked the jacket, so she bought it and added a decorative patch over the hole and another at the lapel height on the front of the garment. The only comment she ever heard was from a gentleman in Colorado who collected patches and wondered where she'd gotten hers and what it stood for. She's worn the jacket about fifteen years now.

Decorative trim covers a multitude of mistakes, redoes, rips, tears, and holes. Visit your fabric store's trim area and let your creative juices flow.

Lapels

Perhaps nothing shows the age of a garment the way an outdated lapel can. Lapels can be restyled, but unless you are a very proficient seamstress, you will need to take the garment to a tailor. Since tailoring is expensive, you would not want a tailor working on an inexpensive garment. If the garment is not worn, is of good quality, and you like it, consider having the lapels narrowed.

You can also remove lapels entirely. Take the collar and lapels off a garment and turn it into a cardigan-styled jacket. Cut on one side from just above the top buttonhole around to the center back of the neck of the garment. Use that piece as a guide to cut off the other lapel so that both sides match. Then stitch about ¼ inch from the raw edge to hold everything together. Finish the raw edge with fold-over braid for heavy garments or a decorative bias trim for lighter-weight garments. Sometimes this remodel results in a garment that is more interesting than the original.

Taking In and Letting Out Pants

Jo and her husband recently cleaned out his wardrobe. He had complained about not having enough slacks to wear to work. Jo was skeptical because there seemed to be a fair number of pants hanging on his side of the closet. They were both right. Three pairs of the slacks hanging there were quality wool dress slacks that had not been worn in a while because they were a little snug. These particular slacks had never been enlarged before, so they had plenty of room in the back seam for Jo to let them out. It only took a few minutes with her seam ripper and sewing machine. Now Al is wearing them to work.

Tailored men's pants have a large seam in the back for taking in and letting out. This will accommodate a modest increase in waist size. Of course, you can only let them out the amount of fabric you have in that seam, and if you take them in too much, the pants will not look good or fit right around the hips.

To change the seam size, take out the inside of the waistband (called the facing) first, then increase or decrease the seam size. Then fold down the waistband, lightly steam press it, and re-attach it.

Cuffed slacks can be lengthened by utilizing the extra fabric in the cuff. You will need to carefully remove the stitching, press out the cuff's creases, and measure for the new length. To put in a hem that is about one inch in depth, you may need to trim off some excess fabric and finish the raw edges so they will not unravel.

Flared slacks can be made narrower. To begin, take out the seams from the hem to the knees on both sides of the pants legs. Measure the width of some pants you like. Make that the new width for the pants you are restyling by widening the seam. Widen it the same amount on either side. That will keep the crease in the same place. If you widen only one seam, the crease will be off center. Before you trim off the extra fabric or put the hem back in, try on the pants to make sure you like the results.

Jeans are nearly impossible to restyle or adjust to fit. We think it is much easier to just buy them to fit. They cannot be altered because of the seam construction. Most of our sewing machines cannot handle the thickness of two or three layers of denim fabric. Jeans can be shortened, but that's about it.

Pullovers to Cardigans

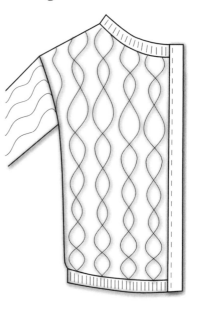

Do you have too many pullover sweaters when what you really need is a cardigan or two? You can turn a pullover sweater into a cardigan. Find the exact center of the front of the pullover. Mark the full length of it with pins or basting stitches. Stitch two rows of stitching ¼ inch apart down the center front of the sweater. That will keep the fabric from unraveling. Cut between the rows of stitching. Now you have the beginning of a cardigan. Cut two pieces of one-inch wide grosgrain ribbon the length of the center of the sweater plus one inch. Stitch the grosgrain ribbon to the sweater by placing the ribbon on the outside and stitching along the edge. Be sure to cover the stitches you made previously. Turn the ½ inch of ribbon at the top and bottom over the edges. Pin in place. Turn the ribbon "facing" to the inside and bond with a fusible web or sew the facing in place. You can also add decorative trim down the front and around the collar if you choose.

Updating Coats

Coats are expensive items, so it makes sense to take care of them and stretch their wearability as long as possible. Mend rips in the coat's lining as soon as they occur. Coat buttons are expensive. Jo tightens coat buttons right away when they become loose, before they fall off and get lost.

A friend of ours thought he needed a new black wool overcoat because the lining of his had come apart in several places. Craig was tired of his arm slipping into the wrong hole. His new bride, Kat, who watches their budget carefully, introduced him to the concept of fixing what you have instead of replacing it. For much less than the price of a new overcoat, this young couple was able to have the coat professionally relined. The coat now has many more years of wear before it needs to be replaced.

If you have a favorite coat and the outside is in good condition but the lining is worn out, you can reline the coat yourself. To do so, take out the lining and carefully take it apart to create a pattern. Then cut a new lining from a good quality lining fabric. Sew it back together in the same way the first lining was put together and sew it back into the coat.

If you are relining a coat instead of buying a new one, you might think about a lining that really adds pizzazz. Get a stripe or a plaid fabric or a truly sumptuous satin lining. Once again, if it all seems too much for you to handle, do what our newlyweds did and get a seamstress to replace the lining. It will be far cheaper than buying a new coat.

Another quick way to update an old coat is to add imitation fur collar and cuffs. Just pick a fake fur that appeals to you, cut it using the coat collar as a pattern, and tack it to the coat collar by turning in the edges of the fur and stitching the new collar to the coat collar all around the edges. To prevent the upper collar from becoming puckered or askew, start at the center back of the collar and stitch around to the front on one side, then go back to the center and stitch the other way to the front. Cuffs are simply straight pieces of fabric cut the diameter of the sleeve plus ½ inch for the seam. Tack these on the same way you would apply the collar—by turning under raw edges and using tiny stitches to hold the cuffs in place.

One more quick change is to change the buttons on the coat. Even though coat buttons are expensive, they will cost less than a new coat. Watch for button sales or closeouts. Sometimes fabric stores put loose buttons into a tub and you can pick out a set of buttons for a minimal cost. Digging through the tub is like a treasure hunt.

All this creative restyling and updating will not only give you and your children more clothing but will also teach them the value of using and reusing what we have. We have more ideas about passing along shoestring clothing to our kids in a later chapter.

Shoestring Tips

1. Notice that sometimes the only difference between an ordinary garment and a designer garment is the embellishments that have been added to the designer garment. You can add these touches to personalize a garment and make it look as though it came from the most expensive shop in town. Shop in those places to see which trims, appliqués, sequins, beading, decorative stitches, buttons, and bows make the difference.

2. While you are in those expensive shops, check out the price tags. That should be enough to send you to a resale store! Gwen recently shopped for a special dress to wear for her son's wedding. She found what she wanted with an eight hundred dollar price tag. She just could not spend it. Gwen then remembered she had seen a lovely dress with an I. Magnin tag on it at a shoestring source. It had been priced at five dollars. It so happens that she gets a senior discount at this particular shoestring place and also had filled out a survey that brought a further discount. The dress ended up costing $1.75. Gwen brought it home,

remodeled the sleeves, and had it dry-cleaned. Since she had previously picked up a pair of nice shoes that just happened to match, she added beautiful stockings and pearl earrings and necklace and went to the special occasion feeling like a million bucks—and looking it too.

3. Sew sequins or set in rhinestones on plain-Jane garments to add pizzazz if that is your style.

4. Add hand embroidery to collars and the fronts of clothing for a personalized look.

5. Learn how to make fabric flowers and use them to embellish dresses at the throat, on scarves, and at the side or middle of the back at the waistline.

6. Make simple berets and long scarves to dress up winter costumes.

7. Add a ruffled or flared overskirt of lace, tulle, or other sheer fabrics to your basic dress.

8. Check out the accessory section of a pattern book.

9. Make a tunic by cutting off a dress at fingertip length and wearing it over a skirt.

10. Cover up a problem or add style to a garment with fabric paints, stenciled-on designs, pom-poms, or buttons sewn in a flower design.

TEN

LET'S GET ORGANIZED

Ted and Bruce Frazzle have a very short to-do list today. It reads, "Organize Bruce's closet and dresser." They do not want to do it. But Ted knows it must be done and looks forward to spending quality time with his son. His positive attitude will eventually rub off on Bruce. And Sally has promised a lasagna dinner if they get it done by mid-afternoon. The guys are motivated.

Since Sally's last rampage through everyone's wardrobes, only things that Bruce actually wears need to be dealt with. Now the guys just have to decide how to best organize it.

The clothing that Bruce wears most often is jeans and T-shirts. These things need to be readily accessible so Bruce can easily find something to wear each day. With this in mind, the T-shirts are hung together in his closet next to his one dress shirt and one casual shirt, which Sally insists are needed now and then. Bruce and Ted hang the T-shirts where they will be most accessible and they hang the other shirts near the back of the closet. That was easy.

Now for the pants. Bruce's one pair of dress pants needs to be hung on a pants hanger so when he needs them they will be wrinkle free and looking good. The other pants in his wardrobe are two pairs of jeans and two pairs of warm-up pants. The easiest way to store jeans is to neatly fold them and put them on shelves that Bruce can reach with ease. For tall Bruce, almost all shelves fall into that category, but shelves at his eye level and just below are easiest to see and deal with. Unfortunately, his closet only has one shelf above the hanging rod. A tower of shelves would come in handy here. And so would bins to hold all the other stuff that needs to be stored on shelves. A trip to the neighborhood hardware store is in order.

The guys are overwhelmed with the wide variety of closet-organizing options available. The bewildered looks on their faces attract the attention of a helpful employee who gives them advice. Ted mentions his tight budget and then says that he has a pretty good idea about how big the closet is. (He should have measured before leaving the house.) The guys purchase a nice white wire closet organization kit. It has a lot of shelves and double-decker rods for hanging clothing. They also purchase a few clear bins that will fit on the shelves.

Back home, Ted and Bruce work together to assemble the new closet organizer. When they are finished they stand back and view their work. The unit looks so nice and clean. Bruce rehangs his shirts and slacks.

Bruce stacks his jeans on the shelf that is easiest to get to and the warm-ups on the shelf just below. His sweatshirts go on the next shelf below that. If they put much more than two or three things in a stack, the stack will quickly become a mess the first time Bruce looks for a particular shirt or pair of jeans. Ted has learned to keep low stacks of clothes in his own closet and now shares this tidbit of wisdom with his son.

A few miscellaneous items also need to be stored. Bruce enjoys participating in sports, so his knee pads, gloves, and so forth are organized on the remaining shelves in clear containers.

Now they tackle the dresser. They empty every drawer, turn the drawers over, and pound on them to remove any crud hiding in the corners of the drawer. This is their way of dusting the drawers, and it is good enough for them! Who is going to see inside their dresser drawers anyway?

They sort the contents of the drawers into piles. There are pajamas, briefs, athletic socks, and shorts. There are also sports-related garments like swim trunks and biking shorts.

They make a nice pile of matching white socks and put them in a top drawer. Every sock is exactly the same, so Bruce can just pull out any two and know they will match. The stack of briefs goes in the same top drawer. A divider between the socks and briefs would be nice but the guys don't think of that. Their eyes are on the clock and lasagna sounds so good.

Pajamas go into the second drawer. They don't fold them, though they should. The guys agree that no one is ever going to see them anyway. The rest of the stuff is loosely organized and placed in the remaining drawers. Bruce has plenty of room to spare since all the outgrown stuff was cleaned out a couple of weeks ago.

Ted and Bruce look around the room to make sure they have taken care of everything. They do not see the bits of crud that fell out of the drawers and need to be vacuumed. They only see that all the clothing has been organized. Bruce should be able to keep it up without too much trouble. It is 2:30 P.M. They can almost taste that lasagna.

If the Frazzle guys can get organized, we know you can as well. Your situation may not be as simple as Bruce's because your wardrobe will most likely be a lot more varied. But the same principles will apply. And we have lots of ideas to get you organized no matter what your situation may be.

Our goal for clothing organization is to make sure everything you use on a daily basis can be found in a moment. This is so important for people who have to go to work, school, or other early morning obligations. One of the ways we ensure this ease of use is by organizing the clothes in our closets by colors and clothing types. All the tops go together and all white blouses hang together, as do blue blouses and so forth. Jo separates her husband's dress shirts from his casual shirts to make it even easier for him on weekday mornings. Our black skirts hang together next to the tan skirts and so on. The slacks are arranged by color together. When Gwen chooses navy blue slacks and wants a red shirt to go with them, she can quickly choose the pants and then, instead of pawing through dozens of blouses and tops, she can go right to the red tops and make her selection from a few pieces. When Jo's husband, Al, gets ready for the office, he chooses a pair of pants from the slacks section, a dress shirt from the dress shirt section, and a matching tie from the tie rack attached to the back of the bedroom door. The matching socks will be found in his sock drawer where Jo keeps his dress socks separate from his athletic socks. Yes, Al is spoiled a little bit, but mornings at the Janssen home are sure pleasant!

Accessories need to be well organized for speedy, stress-free dressing as well. Gwen put up a narrow board—left over from some home decorating project—to organize her scarves. To this board she hot glued a dozen spring-type clothespins spaced evenly along the board with the "mouth" of the clothespins facing downward. She pinches her decorative scarves into the clothespins so that when she wants a particular silk scarf, it is in plain view. Since it has not been folded in some drawer, it is not wrinkled.

Use belt organizers to hold your belts. No one says you have to fit all your belts on just one organizer. You may need several.

Organizers are cheap and will save you loads of time. However, if you or your husband only have two or three belts, it may be easier to attach a hook to the inside wall of your closet to hang them on. A hook-type belt holder can also hold necklaces. It keeps them accessible, prevents them from becoming tangled, and makes it easy to choose the one you want.

If you refit your closet with double rods in part of the closet, you will get twice as much space. Use low rods for your child's current clothing so he or she can reach the clothing and can also put it away easily. You also have room for a lot of storage space over hanging rods in a closet. Most closets have at least one shelf. If there is room, you may be able to fit in an additional shelf above the existing one. The top shelf will be pretty high, so use it for truly off-season clothing and think about buying a small folding stepstool just for your closet.

Shelves come in handy for things that store better folded but are too bulky to fit well into drawers. This might include sweaters, sweat suits, jeans, and work pants. Remember Ted's tidbit of wisdom: More than three things stacked up can quickly turn into a mess. You could place free standing shelves in the closet, but a better alternative might be to install a whole new closet organizer that includes not only a section of shelves but also double-decker rods so you get more hanging space. A handy guy could design and build his own custom closet. There are lots of closet systems available at home improvement stores. Save your money and wait for a sale.

Shoes can be organized in any number of ways. Do not let muddy, greasy, or dirty shoes enter your bedrooms. They need to be cleaned first so other things do not get dirtied. Shoes and boots that are always dirty can be stored near the back door, in a mudroom, or in the garage where they will not spread their grime onto clean clothing. The least expensive closet shoe storage solution is a cardboard shoe holder with a number of slots for your shoes. A visit to a home improvement store will unveil many more shoe organizing options. You may want to free up closet space by hanging a shoe organizer on the back of the closet or bedroom door. A bunch of clear plastic boxes or a wire shoe rack might suit you better.

The other place we usually store clothing is in dresser drawers. And if you are like a lot of our friends, those drawers are not a pretty sight. Jo had to help a friend's son find some clean clothes once while she was baby-sitting him. She could hardly open the dresser drawers because they were so stuffed with clothing. The drawers were a jumbled mess of things the mom had gotten for a song at thrift stores and yard sales. Jo tried to piece together an outfit that looked like it matched. It was difficult because nothing matched. It was the biggest jumble of unmatched pieces of different sized clothing you ever saw. Does that sound familiar?

Sometimes family clothing gets stuffed—or should we say crammed and jammed—into drawers so tightly that it comes out wrinkled. Your spouse and children cannot find clothing items. Emptying the drawer is like working on an archaeological dig. You unearth the complete history of your wardrobe. This is not a good thing! What is the use of having a lot of clothing if you cannot find the piece you are looking for or if it looks awful when you do?

We suggest you remove the contents of all your dresser drawers at least twice a year and get rid of things you are no longer wearing. The first time you do this you may find things you have been missing or have forgotten about. You might have worn some of those things if they had not been shoved in the back of the drawer.

Go through every item and analyze it as you did for your closet. Are you storing rarely used items in your drawers? Consider storing them elsewhere to free up space here in your dresser. Perhaps a well-marked box in a linen closet or under the bed will work.

Now neatly fold everything that is left and put it all in piles on your bed. You will be able to see how much of everything you have so you can figure out how to make the best use of the limited number of dresser drawers available to you. You may be able to put all your underwear and socks in one drawer. You may need two or three drawers. Use the top drawers for the things you use most and the bottom drawers for things that are used less frequently.

Small boxes or dividers that fit into your drawers may help your smaller items stay in one place. Jo puts all of her hosiery in an open-topped box in her lingerie drawer because that slick hosiery tends to shift around and get mixed up in the other things in the drawer. She likes to use clear storage boxes or shoe boxes covered in pretty contact paper. If you are handy, you can build nice dividers for your drawers to help keep things in place.

Kids seem to have the worst time keeping their dressers tidy. You may want to let them use only the drawers they can reach for storing clothing they are currently using. Be patient and keep showing them how to open the drawers completely to put things away neatly and in their correct places. You might need to make sure they do not stuff a whole pile of T-shirts, socks, and underwear into the first drawer that they pull open in their hurry to just get things put away. Since our kids tried that, we assume yours might too.

When you go through your children's dresser drawers, have them help. They may learn a lesson or two. And they may find some treasures they will be glad to see again. Just keep your sense of humor and remember that they are not responsible adults yet, so you should not expect them to be.

Now that every family member can see everything that is in their closets and can even locate their favorite socks and T-shirts in their drawers, you can begin thinking about mixing and matching those coordinated wardrobes to make new outfits.

Mix and Match

You can create new outfits using the same old stuff by remixing what you have and perhaps inserting a couple new things into the old wardrobe collection. A skirt and blouse that was handed down as a matched set may look sadly dated by the time it reaches your family. But if you put the blouse with a skirt that is up-to-date or add a jacket to the whole set, you may come up with a new look that is fresher and more stylish.

To begin the whole process of remixing your wardrobe, go shopping. See what's new in the stores that may already be hiding in your family closets. How is the new style worn? How are pieces paired up? Would you still be able to wear a lot of what you had if you would just wear it differently? Are scarves the rage? Blouses tucked in or out? Sleeves rolled up or left down? How wide are belts? What accessories make an outfit look up-to-date? Check out skirt lengths and silhouettes, jacket lengths, pant lengths and widths, widths of collars and ties, and colors. What kinds of prints and fabrics are being used? Make notes on how to make what you have work with the new way of wearing things and new styles. (You are carrying a small notebook with your needs and sizes listed, right?)

A skirt from a suit may still be usable while you put away the matching jacket until its hopelessly wide lapels come back into style. If your wardrobe is coordinated, that suit skirt will go with other jackets, blouses, and sweaters. A good way to make two separates seem to coordinate beautifully is to wear a scarf or blouse that has colors from both things. So that skirt we mentioned above, in royal blue, paired with a rich red jacket will look great if you find a print blouse that has both royal blue and red in it. The reds and blues do not have to be an exact match but close enough to bring all the pieces together. Or wear a white blouse with the blue skirt and red jacket, and tie a red and royal blue print scarf around your neck.

Your whole family can successfully play the mix-and-match game. Just follow our mix-and-match rules:

1. A wool skirt or dress slacks requires a wool jacket. A linen skirt or dress pants requires a linen jacket. Same with cotton, rayon, silks, and so forth. The weights should be similar as well.

2. You can pair any kind of classic hip-length jacket with blue denim jeans.

3. A casual outfit should be completely casual, a dressy outfit completely dressy. A silky shell meant to be worn with a suit will not look good paired with a pair of canvas shorts.

4. Everything must fit and be in good repair. Clothing should be cleaned and pressed. Bags, shoes, and belts must also be in good repair.

5. You cannot wear very dressy things such as a pinstriped dress jacket from a suit, dressy silky shell, or dressy shoes with cotton khaki pants. Khaki slacks are casual and can only be dressed up so much! A wool, linen, or cotton blazer works. A cotton, rayon, or casual silk top works. Loafers, brogues, and oxfords work. Khaki pants were meant to be paired with sweaters, knit tops, cotton shirts, and golf shirts.

6. Do not mix prints, stripes, and plaids unless you really know what you are doing (that means you have a degree in clothing design or art) or are on your way to a costume party.

7. Before a family member goes out in a new mix-and-match ensemble, have that person try it all on, including socks or hose, shoes, and other accessories. Make sure the outfit looks good and is comfortable and that the wearer can wear it with confidence. Have him or her walk around, sit down, check out all views in a full-length

mirror, and reach up in the air to make sure the outfit is completely comfortable. Check to make sure that nothing pulls or sags, that the skirt or pants are the right length, and that the outfit works with the shoes you have chosen. Make sure the top does not easily come untucked. Take your time and minutely check every detail. After you've done this checking once, the outfit will not need to be checked again. You'll know the pieces go together well and look great. Your family member does not want any embarrassing surprises while wearing this outfit. If you're still not sure, get the opinion of a trusted friend.

8. Make sure you have the correct undergarments for this new ensemble. And make sure they are clean, fit correctly, and are in good repair. No part of a person's undergarments should ever be visible. We really do not want to see the top of your son's briefs, your daughter's bra strap, or your slip hanging below your dress. But if any of those things do accidentally slip into view, at least they should look good. If your slip is torn, the outline of the tear will show through your dress or skirt. Panties that climb will leave a telltale line across your backside. If your daughter has a long, sheer skirt, make sure she also has an adequate slip to go under the outfit.

9. Winter clothing goes with winter clothing; summer clothing goes with summer clothing. Heavy wool pants worn with a sleeveless cotton shirt will not look right.

10. As much as possible, save warm and cool clothing for the right season or weather. People used to follow rather strict rules regarding wearing summer clothing only from Easter to Labor Day. We don't follow those rules anymore, but it is still best to save summer clothing for

warm weather and heavy woolen clothing for winter weather.

11. Tight knit pants are meant to be worn with tops that cover the bottom. They show every dimple, roll, and bulge that most of us prefer to hide and no one else really wants to see.

12. A man can use a solid-colored jacket from a suit to mix with other slacks, but never a pinstripe suit jacket.

13. It is easier to mix and match solid-colored items than prints, so take a more serious look at the hand-me-downs that are not prints, checks, or stripes. Solid colors also have more longevity in the fashion world. Prints go out of style sooner. Solids are less memorable so can be worn more frequently than prints that catch the eye.

14. Arrange your closet so all the pants are together, the shirts are together, and so on. It is quicker and easier to mix and match and see what you have when your closet is organized.

15. Lay out all of one person's clothing in a room and try different pieces together. Some experts suggest you make a list of all the possible combinations and hang it near the closet.

This may all seem like a lot of trouble just to save a few dollars. We do not think so. The process also increases your creative abilities. We enjoy the challenge. Rather than spending the time looking for just the right dress, we could have saved a lot of time and money by making something we already own work for the special occasion.

You really do want to save money. And if you use our money-saving ideas consistently, they will become habits. Hopefully your children will pick up on the same shoestring habits that you are developing.

Shoestring Tips

1. Be picky. You want to look good, not cheap. Having a few good things is much better than having a bunch of junky things.

2. Spend some time at the mall to learn how your old clothing can be paired with other items to create new looks.

3. Spend a couple of hours in the library perusing fashion magazines to help you keep up with the new styles.

4. Give yourself a complete, head-to-toe critical look before going out the door each day, especially when wearing a new mix of clothing. You don't want to look like you got dressed in the dark.

5. Do some people watching. Pretend to be the clothing police. Take notes on what looks good and what looks tacky.

6. Be daring. Have fun.

7. When evaluating something, try it on with the correct undergarments and shoes. Button every button, zip up the zippers, and tie the ties to get a true analysis.

8. Look in a full-length mirror, and also use a hand mirror to get a rear view.

9. Check out your local home improvement or hardware stores for ideas and materials to better organize your closets.

10. Go to the library for how-to books if you want to build your own closet system. (Using the library saves money too.)

11. Add hooks to the back of doors for hanging bathrobes or other bulky items.

12. Hang a tie rack on the back of a door to make it easy to find and get the right tie.

13. Organize a man's ties by colors.

14. Find another place to store dressy clothing such as suits and dresses if they are rarely used. That way they will not clog up your closet. Or at least put them in the hardest to reach part of the closet. A rack in the basement, the guest room closet, or other spare space may work. Just be sure to keep clothing protected from dust and moths.

15. Periodically check drawers, closets, and shelves in your kids' rooms to make sure things are being properly stored. Help your kids out a bit if necessary.

16. Put things where they belong. You know the saying: "Do it right the first time." It will make finding things so much easier.

ELEVEN

TEACHING YOUR CHILDREN HOW TO DRESS ON A SHOESTRING

Gwen had a lot of trouble convincing her teenage daughter that it was okay to save money on clothing by shopping in thrift shops and discount stores. She had trouble, that is, until one day a model who attended their church gave a seminar and told where she was finding her gorgeous clothes—thrift and resale shops. Now Gwen's teenager is grown and knows all the best shoestring locations in her city. She not only shops the local charity thrift shops but also makes purchases at the trade mart when it is open to the general public. She watches for sales and buys basic mixable clothing. She has her own style and stays with it, thereby limiting the amount of clothes she needs. Gwen taught her well.

We were both fortunate enough to learn the principles of shoestring living from our parents. Neither of us grew up in prosperous environments. Our parents taught us to use and reuse everything, to make something out of nothing, to be content with what we had, and, most importantly, that there are more important things in life than money and the things it can buy. Jo's father, the pastor of a small church, often reminded his family that they were rich in love. And they were.

While our parents struggled to make ends meet while still feeding and clothing a bunch of kids, they were unwittingly teaching us many lessons in frugality. The same opportunity exists for you and your children. The shoestring lifestyle, done with grace and a positive outlook, will be caught, if not necessarily taught.

SCRIPTURAL PRINCIPLES OF GOOD STEWARDSHIP

Certain spiritual truths about good stewardship of resources are the underlying basis of a shoestring lifestyle. The first and hardest one may be that we should practice contentment with what we have. This is difficult in a world that bombards all our senses with advertisements designed to brainwash us into believing we will be happy, loved, popular, and sexy if we own, wear, or use the latest products.

The human desire to be loved and accepted is so strong that we buy the "magic potions," hoping they will help us get the love and acceptance we desire. However, if the need for unconditional love and acceptance is met through our relationship with God and the security of a loving family, then we won't be so attracted by the world's solutions.

If all those ads you come across every day are giving you and your family the "I wannas" and causing discontent, perhaps you all need to wean yourselves from them. They usually enter our lives through TV, magazines, newspaper ads, and window-shopping. Turn off the TV, rip out or ignore the magazine ads, toss the newspaper ads, and find another hobby besides window-shopping. Teach your family to look at advertising with a critical eye and discerning mind.

Secondly, the Bible constantly exhorts us to be wise with our money, not wasting it. This means we live within our budgets and do not frivolously toss money away. Proverbs 11:15; 21:20; and 28:19 encourage us to handle our resources wisely. In the parable of the talents, Jesus admonished his followers to be wise with the gifts and talents our Master has entrusted to us (see Matthew 25).

We really hate to pay full retail prices for anything, but especially clothing. We feel like we are better stewards of our resources when we spend as little as possible. It may take a little more effort to make sure you have found the best price for something you need. But we feel the result is well worth the effort.

Third, never go into debt to clothe your family. Paul warns about debt in Romans 13:8, and you will find more warnings in Proverbs 11:15 and 22:7. Debt can be a never-ending, ever-growing monster that can eat up your emotions, savings, and peace of mind. Do not get caught in its trap. If you cannot afford fifty dollars this month to buy a new blouse, what makes you think you will be able to afford it next month when the credit card bill is due? Will another emergency come up then that will prevent you from paying it off? Children bring a lot of unexpected expenditures. Make sure your budget has leeway for those book orders, snacks for the team, field trips, party gifts, school supplies, and so on.

Fourth, if you are spending more on clothing than you are on tithing to your church, you need to check your priorities and rethink your budget. For Christians, tithing is a must. Second Corinthians 8–9, especially 9:6–13, addresses the subject of giving generously to the church. The opposite of generosity is the spiritual problem of greed, which Jesus talks about at length in Luke 12:15–21, 32–34.

Your spiritual rewards will be greater if you tithe to your church than if you show up in a new outfit every Sunday. We want to lead our families to put their treasures where their hearts are. Your budget and checkbook register give a very good indication of where your heart is. I do not remember any mention in the Bible about spiritual rewards for wearing expensive clothing. And do not forget, your children are watching.

Fifth, God provides for his people. Remember how he adorns the lilies of the field. You do not need to worry about anything, much less what you will wear. Read Matthew 6:19–34 and Philippians 4:4–9 if you need a reminder of God's sovereign loving care of his children.

Sometimes we have to practice patience and contentment while waiting for God to meet our needs. Sometimes the things that we think are needs are really not needs at all. They may be wants or things our selfish pride would very much like to have. Yes, it is nice to have a nice new outfit to wear to church. But is it a need? Are you afraid people will think less of you because you wear the same thing week after week? That is pride.

TEACHING KIDS TO MAKE WISE CLOTHING CHOICES

Begin training your children in wardrobe management as soon as they are able to pick out what they want to wear. First of all, figure out a way to put their clothing down at eye level for them. Use bottom drawers of a bureau for their clothing.

Add drop rods to their closets so that their clothing hangs at eye level. Teach them how to pick tops and bottoms that match.

Just as important as dressing is taking proper care of their clothing. Even little ones can put their dirty things in a handy hamper, and if their closets and drawers are at their level, they can put their things away.

Make living well within your means a fun challenge for the whole family. Talk about what you need to buy, how much you want to spend, and what you will do with any money that is left over. Be open, positive, and creative.

SHOPPING WITH THE FAMILY

Perhaps the best way to teach your kids about shoestring dressing is to take them shopping with you and talk about it while you inspect the merchandise. Think out loud as you go through a rack of sale items. Hold up and inspect different items to teach them lessons. Listen to their opinions about different fashions, colors, and so on. Soon they will begin to look at things critically.

What to Teach Them about Clothing While You Shop

Someday quality will be very important to your children, but they may not see the need when they are young and desperately desire a shirt with their hero on it. Explain that better quality things will last longer. You can also be thinking of the people who will receive the clothing as hand-me-downs. Clothing will last through several kids, still looking good and in good condition, if the quality is good and the style not too trendy. Most superheroes are trendy.

Let your children handle the garments with clean hands so they can get the feel, or "hand," of different fabrics. They will notice that denim comes in different weights. Some knits are tighter and nicer than others. Some fabrics fray more easily, lose their shape, pill, wrinkle easily, or feel uncomfortable on the skin.

Point out the tags and labels sewn into the garments. Note the makeup of the fabric. Let them feel the difference between 100 percent cotton, cotton and polyester blends, and pure polyester. Silk, rayon, nylon, wool, and the many blends have particular characteristics and feel. Note the washing instructions. Find out if something has to be hand washed, dried flat, hung to dry, or dry-cleaned. Mention that it may be more trouble or expense than you want.

Look inside the garments to let your children check out the seam allowance, how the seams are finished, and how well the whole garment is stitched.

Eventually the whole family will recognize that some brands of clothing and shoes are consistently well constructed. Some family members may realize that a certain brand of pants seems to always fit him better than other brands. They will discover that certain brands of shoes can always be counted on to not only wear well but also have adequate room in the toes and good arch supports. While those brands may be very reliable, teach the family to continue experimenting with lesser-known brands as well. Makers continually change the way they style and cut their clothing, so nothing is a sure thing forever.

When shopping to buy, you will not only be teaching your family what to look for but also how to stick to a list. There are many pretty, cool, and new-looking things alluringly displayed to catch your eye. But you have a list and a budget. You can enjoy looking at and admiring all the wonders of the fashion world at your favorite mall, but you must still exercise self-control.

Train yourself and then teach your children to ask if you really need something new before you buy it. Do you already have something that would fill the same slot in your wardrobe that this new item would? Would you really wear it often? Is this an emotional decision? Is it in the budget? Do you have the cash to buy it? Is it on sale?

If you or your child are sure you *must* have this thing, ask the store to hold it for a few hours. Go home, think about it, and inspect your wardrobe to see if you really need it. Ask yourself if this need to buy is a sign of discontentment. If you decide this is really a clothing need and not an emotional need, feel free to return to the store and buy it. But go prepared. Wear whatever you will be wearing with that item. Try it on to make sure it works. Are the pants too short to go with the shoes you planned on wearing? Does your slip show? Does the belt fit through the belt loops? If you need to buy new shoes, hose, belt, undergarments, or something else to match, it might not be such a good buy after all. Remember that your brain cannot accurately remember colors. You must have the clothing item you intend to wear with the new purchase to really match them up right. Teach your children to go through these steps and they will become excellent clothing shoppers who buy out of genuine need and not out of emotional need.

If you will follow these suggestions for yourself, your budget, and your peace of mind and as a way to teach your children how to live on a shoestring, you will all enjoy many benefits and blessings, just like the Frazzle women are about to experience.

Sally Frazzle Shops with Her Daughter

In August advertisers tell us what we need to buy to send our kids back to school. The latest fashions and gadgets are cleverly promoted, geared to convince kids those things are must-haves. Sally and Spacy have been looking at these ads together, trying to cut through the hype to discern what Spacy really requires for her back-to-school wardrobe. Spacy wants to look fashionable. And while Sally wants her daughter to fit in with the other kids at school, budget is her main concern. Sally convinces Spacy to at least try out the local thrift and resale stores before going to the mall for all new clothing. They discuss the limited budget and make a list of Spacy's needs. They seem to be on the right course.

As they begin a Saturday of thrift shopping, Spacy is afraid someone might see her entering a thrift store and make a negative judgment about her. Then she realizes that the only people near the thrift store are other thrift store customers, and she relaxes. Upon entering the first store on the list, she realizes that this might be fun because the first thing that catches her eye is a display of retro stuff that looks kind of cool.

Sally and Spacy quickly find women's clothing and begin to search the racks. They laugh together at some of the outrageous things they find. Spacy finds a blouse just like the one Grandma wears all the time, which evokes fond memories. Sally finds a dress just like the one she wore to a banquet twenty years ago! But amongst all the really old and funny stuff, they also uncover some real bargains. They are amazed that people buy clothing and never wear it, sometimes even leaving the tags on. They find some never worn and hardly ever worn items that are still quite fashionable. After trying a few on and finding a couple of things that just perfectly meet her needs, Spacy is quite enthusiastic about this new shopping experience. She sees how she may get more clothing than she thought possible with her mother's budget.

After a day of thrift shopping and even finding some resale shops that were new to them, the Frazzle girls come home tired but happy. They crossed several items off the list and spent very little money. The garments will need to be laundered, of course, but they all look new, fit well, and are becoming and well made. Sally will have to sew on exactly one button. (Do people really give away clothes just because a button is missing and they do not want to or know how to sew it back on? Yes, as Sally will tell you, they do.)

Spacy could not believe she got so much for so little. And it was fun too. Of course, she will never tell anyone where she found these clothes! Little does she know that many of her friends and acquaintances harbor the same secret.

On another Saturday a couple of weeks before school begins, Sally and Spacy visit the mall to take advantage of the sales. They stick to a set budget and carry a list of Spacy's remaining wardrobe needs. They have learned that it is fun shopping together when both understand the budgetary ground rules. It is almost like a game. They arrive just as the stores are opening.

They begin by visiting every store that carries what they need, writing down in Sally's little notepad the prices, colors, brands, available sizes, and name of the store. They find some great sales and the stores seem to be well stocked with the styles, colors, and sizes that Spacy likes.

Then Sally sees something that is too good to be true. It is a blazer that she simply must have. It is her color, it fits (she knows because she tried it on as soon as she saw it!), it looks marvelous on her, and it will match ten other things hanging in her closet. But it is not on Sally's list. In fact it costs more than she intended to spend on all the other things on Spacy's school clothing list put together.

At this point we must ask ourselves why Sally is flirting so intensely with temptation in the first place! Was she just doing "research" like we taught her? But of course! The problem is, now she is tempted and must think things through. How important are those other things on her list? Spacy would say they are imperative. And she needs to think about what she is teaching Spacy. Maybe she should wait until this perfect garment goes on sale or clearance.

Sally prudently writes down the price and location of this fabulous blazer and returns her focus to her daughter's needs. That was a close call. She nearly blew the budget.

Meanwhile Spacy discovers a pair of jeans that she is sure everyone else at school will be wearing. It was inevitable that she would discover these jeans. The store planned and connived so that every teenage girl in the mall would just happen to notice these cleverly and prominently displayed jeans. Spacy confidently, sincerely, and most definitely must have these jeans. Tears, a protruding lower lip, and Bambi eyes miraculously appear to aid her arguments. What is Sally to do?

What she does *not* do is yell, scream, or even get the least bit angry. After all, *she* just came through a similar spending crisis. Sally calmly reminds Spacy of the agreed-upon list and budget. Then they talk about choices. If Spacy wants the jeans, she will have to give up several other items she wants. Or she could put up her own money to buy the jeans herself. Or she could wait to see if everyone really is wearing these particular jeans at school next week.

Because Sally is an adult, she knows that this will be a learning experience and lets Spacy make her own decision—even if it is a mistake. Will it really do irreparable damage if Spacy has to wear holey socks and last year's coat so she can have her heart's desire of a pair of stylish jeans? Probably not. Will it hurt her social life if she uses all her saved-up "fun money"? Sally doubts it. Spacy will, however, learn that Sally trusts her, is letting her grow up, and loves her no matter what she does with her hard-earned money. And Spacy will probably make wiser decisions next August when she realizes her coat is truly too small and those fancy jeans did not bring her popularity, make her look like a model, or win anyone's heart.

The pair decides to treat themselves to a light lunch while they think it over. On the way to the food court they see the same pair of jeans, 40 percent off, at another store. "Maybe we should check other stores too," says quick-to-learn Spacy. So after they have pizza and a glass of water, they make another round of the stores. It seems that 40 percent off is the best deal on jeans at the mall. Spacy tries on a few pairs in different sizes. One pair fits perfectly. Now she has to decide whether or not to buy them. Spacy decides that she will make up the difference between what her mom intended to spend for a pair of jeans and the price of the jeans. It will mean going to fewer movies with her friends, but she will look for more baby-sitting jobs to earn more spending money later. It is worth it to her to have this pair of jeans. The budget is saved and Spacy is ecstatic.

Amazingly, the Frazzle ladies have a wonderful time shopping together. Spacy only pretended twice, when they saw some girls from school, that she wasn't with her mom. And they were able to find almost everything on their list. Spacy's closet is now full of coordinating items that she can mix and match. They are all becoming to her figure and coloring. Sally even made sure that they were all modest as well. Even though the popular style is to show cleavage, lots of thigh, and the abdomen, they were able to find things that covered all those parts. They will watch the ads for sales on the remaining items on her list.

Other Ways to Handle
the Budget Game with Children

Sally and Spacy went shopping with Sally holding the cash in her wallet. That may not be what works best for every family. Perhaps your children would not be caught dead at a mall with a parent. Perhaps you can trust them to figure out how to make the clothing budget work for themselves.

Recently our friend Vickie's son Trevor informed his mom that he wanted to do his own shopping. If she would give him the cash that she would ordinarily spend in a year on his clothing, he would make it stretch to fill his needs. Since she trusts her thirteen-year-old son, Vickie agreed to his plan.

When it was time to buy clothes, however, he discovered that retail stores eat up cash awfully fast. He asked his mom to take him to some thrift stores where he was able to buy quite a bit more than he needs and have some money left over. He will surely grow over the next twelve months, so Vickie is curious to see how Trevor will deal with future needs. He may end up wearing short pants by next spring. But he will have learned about thinking ahead, about all the items in a wardrobe that we usually forget but need, about delayed gratification, and many other lessons as well.

As kids get older and get jobs, you may require them to help out with their clothing needs. You may offer to buy them a few basics and leave the rest up to them.

Whatever you do, teach your kids that your checkbook, wallet, or credit card is not a bottomless pit. Let them know how much you want to spend. Get them involved with the family budget. They can help you comparison shop and think through their clothing needs.

Every August and March, Jo goes through her kids' wardrobes with them to analyze what they need. Actually, she now lets the boys do their own sorting and analyzing because over the years she has taught them how to do it well. Little Anna still gets some assistance. Jo also has a box of hand-me-downs to go through.

Each child makes a list of needs for the coming season. By starting the fall and winter shopping in August, they will have what they need before the first frost surprises them. In March, during spring break, they think ahead to summer's needs so when school is out and the weather is warm, they are ready.

Jo tells the kids how much she intends to spend for each item. For example, if Jonathan needs four shirts and she wants to spend no more than ten dollars on each shirt, that may mean that if he finds one for five dollars, he can spend fifteen dollars on another. They attack the shopping in true conqueror fashion, searching for the best prices. When they get to the men's department of a store, they spread out to find the best finds. While they are shopping, the kids inform everyone exactly what they will and will not wear. They do not waste their time looking at anything they know the boys will not like. Jo's boys make quick work of buying clothing. Anna could shop for hours every day if she were allowed. Needless to say, the boys' stuff is purchased first and fastest. The girls can go out shopping later without the boys.

Jo recently tried to shop for pants for Jonathan while Jonathan was at school. She thought she knew what size to buy and could save both of them a lot of time and trouble. She was wrong. The pants were way too big around the waist. So Jo and Jonathan had to go shopping together after all. They discovered that he wears 28W x 32L and that there are not very many khaki slacks in his size in town. They eventually found some at a discount store. Jo will not waste her time again buying pants without the kids along to try them on.

Then Jo thought Josh would like the nice Denver Broncos T-shirts she found at Sam's Club. He liked that kind last year and still wears them, she reasoned. Again, she was wrong. He did not get excited about the shirts at all. He thinks he *might* wear them during football season. Jo is still learning to follow her own advice about always taking the kids with her when choosing their clothing.

Every family needs to figure out how to best keep everyone clothed and happy while staying within a budget and teaching the kids how to do the same. Life is too complicated and full of too many temptations to spend money. Our children need our guidance and training before they face the big, expensive world on their own.

Caring for Clothing

When Jo was a little girl, she lost her sweater at school. She never found it. Her parents did not buy her another sweater. She had to do without one for the rest of the winter. Do not feel too sorry for her, though, because she lived in Yuma, Arizona.

She was not suffering from extreme cold and she did have a coat. But she really missed having a sweater. She never again lost another sweater or any other piece of clothing. Her parents let her learn an important lesson.

Her parents also taught her another important lesson. Jo's mother must have said a thousand times, "If you want to be pretty, you have to be nice and neat and clean." She was right, of course. You cannot look good if you or your clothes are dirty or in disrepair.

Since it is so expensive to clothe ourselves, we must take care of what we have. And it is important to teach our kids to take care of what they have as well. Not only do they need to learn to gather all their belongings before leaving a place, but they also need to learn to respect and care for their belongings.

Many of us, adults included, do not care for our things as we should. It is easier, we reason, to toss them out and replace them with new things. This is wasteful and expensive. Our parents had a great idea when they taught us to use, reuse, fix, and recycle everything. We should come back to that thinking.

Our children need to know that clothing will not be thrown out when it needs repair. They need to be aware that when their clothing needs repair, we can do something about it. A stitch in time really does save nine. They also need to let us know about spills, stains, and spots. The sooner those are dealt with, the better. Teach your kids to let you know when there is a problem with their clothing. If they have not worn something for a while, ask them if there is something wrong with it.

Your kids will be afraid to show you their rips and stains if they are sure they will receive an angry response. Let them know that they are safe from punishment if they are hard on their clothing as long as they are not doing anything intentionally destructive. In fact, healthy little kids will be hard on their clothing if they are as active as they should be. Jo did put her foot down, though, when she caught one of her sons using the toes

210

of his sneakers for slowing himself on his bicycle. That is what brakes are for!

On the other hand, kids do need to learn that when they are dressed up, they need to act dressed up. They will not be running around and playing rough when they are wearing better clothing. Be fair to your kids by only requiring them to wear dressy things for limited times and special occasions. They can only be so good and so quiet for so long, you know. Do not expect adult behavior from little people. And do not give them red drinks and other stuff that stains. That's asking for trouble!

Part of respecting our property is not treating it destructively. Children must learn that using their sneakers for bicycle brakes, wiping up spills with their clothing, and other such behavior is destructive and will not be allowed. Be patient. They don't know about these things unless they are warned, taught, and told—sometimes repeatedly.

Even very young kids can learn how to soak out mud stains, show you their grass stains, and point out their missing buttons and holes. Do not be too dismayed about stains. Just deal with them right away. At a nearby fabric store we found specialized stain removers for just about every conceivable stain: colors that have run, fat, grease, oil, fruit, red wine, ink, rust, ketchup and sauces, grass, clay, chewing gum, glue, tea/coffee/cola, and even crayon.

Kids can also begin learning how to sew on buttons, sort laundry, and fold small items of clothing. Matching socks is a good prereading exercise, and folding them up into sock balls strengthens the little fingers that are learning to write. You are never too early or too late to teach your kids how to do laundry, ironing, and mending.

You may have to post written instructions in your laundry room to help the children remember everything. It can be confusing at first. Some families have each person sort his or her laundry before putting it in the laundry room. They have three labeled baskets or bins of some kind for sorting. Set aside certain days for laundry so your family knows when to have everything in one of the laundry piles. This lets them know when to expect something back out of the laundry as well. (How many more days do I have to wear these dirty socks?)

We recommend waiting until a child is eight or older to begin teaching the art of ironing. Ironing makes it so easy to burn oneself. Or scorch a shirt. Or burn the house down. Begin lessons with easy things like table napkins and handkerchiefs. With plenty of supervision, move to clothes without too many buttons, plackets, and other details. Jo's daughter practiced on her doll's clothing. Teach them about temperatures, steam, spraying, starching, and hanging things up neatly afterwards. They will eventually need to learn how to use a pressing cloth for woolens, how to iron fabrics like corduroy from the inside, and how to iron neat creases in slacks.

As we mentioned before, make sure your kids have adequate and easy-to-reach storage for their clothing. This helps them keep it neat and encourages them to put away their own clothing. If a drawer is too full, the clothing will not stay neatly folded. If the closet bar is too high, the clothing cannot be hung up. Do a daily check of their bedrooms to make sure everything is properly put away. Occasionally work with them to clean out drawers and closets to eliminate overcrowding.

Your kids won't have much of an excuse for leaving dirty clothing around if there is a hamper or laundry basket handy. If clothing does not land in the dirty clothes hamper, do not wash it. After your child is out of clean clothes and you point out the reason, he will learn to put his dirty clothing in the hamper. It will not do permanent harm if a child wears dirty socks for a day or two. He can always do his own load of laundry or wash things by hand. Washing things may need some control later on when teenagers want to run to the washing machine to wash one or two items. That's expensive and a waste of electricity, water, and soap. Teach them to run full loads.

Show your children how to properly hang up different types of garments. It may be hard for them to learn to do it neatly. It may be easier if they lay the clothing item out flat on a bed while trying to get it on a hanger properly. Be patient; this is a lot more difficult for kids than it sounds.

Have you ever seen someone who is impeccably dressed except that his or her shoes are not shined? It ruins the whole effect! We have met people who actually judge a person's character on whether or not that person's shoes are shined. That may be overdoing it, but attention to detail is important.

When your teenagers begin wearing nice dress shoes, give them some shoe trees so they can learn to care for their shoes properly. Teach them to polish their shoes and warn them about too much moisture (you know, from walking in puddles and such) harming their good shoes. Shoes that have gotten dirty need to be cleaned right away. That way they will be ready for the next time they are needed and the dirt is not spread in the closet.

Shoes that are not worn very often should be stored in such a way that they do not get dusty. Hanging shoe bags or clear plastic boxes will work. Some people keep all their shoes in the shoe boxes they came in, neatly stacked on the closet floor.

In short, just in case your kids do not pick up on your good clothing-care habits, make it a point to train them. They may not see you caring for your clothing when you are behind a closed bedroom door or in the laundry room. We cannot be sure they know things unless we have methodically taught them and checked on them.

Again, remember that kids must be kids. I would worry about a little boy who did not get holes in the knees of his play pants. Little people fall down, spill things, and are uncoordinated and sloppy. A lot of adults are as well! This is part of life and to be expected. Learn how to remove stains and do some mending, and you will be able to be a lot more even tempered when accidents happen.

ONE LAST SALLY FRAZZLE STORY

On a beautiful summery Friday morning in September, our friend Sally awakes to the chirping of birds and a jackhammer destroying the street in front of her house. Oh well. It was time to get up, anyway.

Sally follows her usual morning routine: a quiet time, a hot shower, a yogurt and granola breakfast, and then the usual application of cosmetics before facing her closet to find something to wear. Some people decide the night before. Sally has not come that far yet.

Her newly organized closet is a delight. All her slacks hang together and are grouped by color on the higher of the two rods in this part of her closet. Next to the pants are her skirts, with the tan ones next to the brown ones next to her green one. On the rod below are her blouses and blazers, all organized by color as well. Her dresses and longer skirts hang in the next section. Her shoes hang in a shoe bag. This is a huge improvement over the shoe jumble that used to clutter her closet floor.

There are so many choices this morning. It helps that she spent last Saturday mending. And Spacy is doing a good job of keeping up on the laundry. What shall she wear?

The tan suit skirt no longer hangs in her closet, but the suit jacket does. There are several attractive options for what to wear with the jacket. Sally does the eeny-meeny-miney-mo thing, then pulls some brown slacks from the closet. Now for a top. Hmmm. The weather forecast calls for a cool morning but an afternoon high of 75 degrees. A cream-colored golf shirt will work. Sally pulls a brown belt from the hanging belt rack and finds her brown loafers in the shoe rack. When she has finished dressing, she inspects herself in the full-length mirror. Sally is pleased with the total effect.

Apparently Ted likes the total effect too, as he comes up behind his attractive wife to give her a quick squeeze. He smiles at the two of them reflected in the mirror.

Ted feels confident to face the day—he has a presentation to make—in his new gray suit. With a freshly ironed white shirt, conservative power tie, and shined wing tips, he looks as good as he feels—ready to conquer the business world.

Down the hall Spacy can be heard wailing, "I can't decide what to wear!" She has tried on a dozen outfits and they all look good. She cannot decide which one to wear today.

In the previous months, Spacy has learned that she has a style—Artsy-Creative, actually—and that she has "summer" coloring. Armed with that knowledge, she has removed from her closet and drawers all the things that do not look good on her and has begun collecting becoming clothing. Thanks to her new thrifting hobby, she has lots of clothing choices.

While looking like her peers is still important to her, she is readjusting her priorities. Two things influenced that. First, the whole family went on a short missions trip to Mexico. They returned very thankful for their prosperous lifestyle. Second, her parents took her and Bruce out of the youth group for what seemed to them like a *really* long time (four weeks) to attend a money management class. They were the only two kids in the adult class. Spacy was *so* embarrassed. But it did help get the family's budget back on track.

Just before she has to run to catch the school bus, Spacy pulls on a bright pink top and some blue jeans. Frantically she looks in her jewelry box for something to go with the top. She grabs some earrings her brother made for her as a birthday gift. She had no idea he even noticed things like jewelry fashions, much less had the ability to make something so nice that was so *her*.

That surprisingly thoughtful big brother had also learned a few things lately. Bruce found a part-time job doing janitorial work on weekends at a business complex two blocks away. He is learning to save his money for important things like college. In fact, he purchased the coveted Magic Marvel High-Top Springfoot Basketball Shoes with his own hard-earned cash.

He emerges from his bedroom wearing a clean pair of jeans, a T-shirt with no wrinkles in it ("Space," as he calls his sister, has been hanging up his shirts when they come out of the dryer), and of course his new basketball shoes. He looks pretty good and feels pretty good as well. After all, he looks like a shoe-in (pun intended) for the varsity basketball team, and some colleges are interested in him.

The Frazzles find that some things are running smoother these days. And not just because they are all able to find something to wear every morning. They are all growing spiritually as they learn the importance of tithing and using their resources wisely. The short mission trip they took over the Christmas holidays showed them how richly blessed and prosperous they really are. Living on a shoestring has become a challenging family game that is actually kind of fun. Every day they count their blessings.

Shoestring Tips

1. Discuss the realities of your budget with your children. You will be surprised how quickly they catch on.

2. Check out library books about clothing construction, personal style, and stain removal.

3. Have a thankful heart. Remind yourself and your family members what you *do* have—all gifts from God!

4. Start a clothing exchange in your church, school, or neighborhood.

5. Only carry and spend cold, hard cash when shopping with your kids. When it is gone, it is gone.

6. Give your kids an allowance and some training in handling it.

7. Check out the library for books about teaching your kids to handle money.

8. Make sure each family member knows what styles and colors look best on him or her.

9. Organize each person's closets and chest of drawers to make it easier to put things away properly and to retrieve them easily. Make a place for everything and keep everything in its place.

10. Teach your children how to sew, or send them to someone who can teach them.

11. Read Mary Hunt's *Debt-Proof Your Kids*.

12. Give your kids their own lint remover.

13. Learn to clean white leather shoes with old-fashioned white toothpaste (not the gel type). There is just enough fine grit in the toothpaste to cut through black marks on white shoes without scratching the leather.

14. Practice delayed gratification, contentment, and generosity in front of and with your family.

15. Meditate on Matthew 6:25–34.

16. Enjoy having a really nicely dressed family—all on a shoestring!

GLOSSARY

A-line skirt. A skirt with a straight flare from waist to hem.

appliqué. Designs or decorations applied on fabric or the process of applying them.

basting stitches. Long stitches used when sewing to temporarily hold things together.

bias cut. Cut of garment in which the threads in the material run on the diagonal instead of straight up and down or across.

bolt of fabric. A long length of fabric rolled onto a cardboard rectangle or tube; the most common way fabric is stored and displayed in fabric stores.

brooch. A large decorative pin or clasp.

coatdress. A dress that has no seam at the waistline and buttons down the front like a coat.

consignment shops. Shops that sell used goods and share the profit with the consignee.

core wardrobe. A collection of well-coordinated pieces, usually based on a neutral color, that mix and match with each other and meet the needs of the wearer for most occasions.

dickey. A blouse front with only the collar and a bit of fabric around the collar to tuck into the garment being worn; takes the place of a shirt or blouse under a sweater, with a suit, or with a low-necked garment.

family lifestyle. A description of how your family really lives. In this book lifestyles are classified as Metropolitan, Middle American, or Casual. Your particular family's lifestyle may be a combination of two or more of these styles.

fusible hemming tape. Iron-on tape that eliminates the need to sew a hem.

gabardine. A twill weave of fabric that is extremely tight and durable.

hem gauge. See sewing gauge.

I. Magnin. A high-end retail company known for quality merchandise.

individual style. The style of clothing an individual is most comfortable in. In this book individual styles are classified as Sporty-Casual, Classic, Romantic, High Fashion–Dramatic, and Artsy-Creative. You may be a combination of two or more styles.

khaki. A sturdy cloth that is usually colored light olive to yellowish brown.

Loafer. A trademark for a low leather step-in shoe; commonly used to describe any such shoe.

military braid. Braided trim like that used on military uniforms.

neutral colors. Colors that seem to go with just about anything in a wardrobe, such as black, gray, brown, tan, cream, and white.

patent leather. Black leather finished to a hard, glossy surface; many good imitations of patent leather are made of synthetic materials.

personal style. See individual style.

placket. A slit in a garment to give the wearer ease of movement or to make it easier to get the garment on; often found above a shirt cuff, at the front neckline of a golf shirt, or on a skirt.

proportion. The size of each part in relation to the other parts; in fashion, the human body is imagined to be divided in thirds, and the most attractive styles create a break in style between one of the thirds and the other two thirds, rather than creating two equal lengths.

sewing gauge. A small ruler with a sliding marker to help measure hem depths accurately.

shank button. A button with a stem or shaft on its underside that has a hole in it for attaching the button to a garment.

sheath. A dress that has no seam at the waist and is usually close fitting with narrow, straight lines.

shell. A sleeveless, collarless blouse that is worn under suits or cardigans; can be made of silk, rayon, or cotton.

Shetland wool. A fine, loosely twisted yarn made from the wool of sheep raised in the Shetland Islands; a garment knitted of this wool is warm and lightweight.

shoe trees. A foot-shaped form inserted into shoes to help them keep their shape.

soutache. A narrow, braided clothing trim with a herringbone pattern.

straight grain. Describes a garment with the threads in the fabric running straight up and down and straight across.

transfers. Iron-on designs that can be affixed to fabric.

Wonder-Under. A brand-name adhesive material used to make two layers of fabric adhere to each other; the sheet of material is ironed to activate the adhesive.

RECOMMENDED READING

Albert, Donna. *No-Sew Special Effects: Quilts, Crafts, Clothing, Home Décor.* Radnor, Pa.: Chilton Book Company, 1996.

Bensussen, Rusty. *Sew Your Own Fashion Accessories.* New York: Sterling Publishing, 1990.

Fatt, Amelia. *Conservative Chic.* New York: Times Books, 1983.

Feldon, Leah. *Dressing Rich.* New York: G. P. Putnam's Sons, 1982.

Grimble, Frances, and Deborah Kuhn. *After a Fashion: How to Reproduce, Restore, and Wear Vintage Styles.* San Francisco, Calif.: Lavolta Press, 1998.

Jackson, Carole. *Color Me Beautiful.* New York: Ballantine Books, 1973.

Kleeber, Irene Cumming, ed. *The Butterick Fabric Handbook.* New York: Butterick Publishing, 1975.

Nix-Rice, Nancy, and Pati Palmer. *Looking Good: A Comprehensive Guide to Wardrobe Planning, Color, and Personal Style Development.* Portland, Ore.: Palmer Pletsch Publishing, 1996.

Pooser, Doris. *Always in Style: The Complete Guide for Creating Your Best Look: Style, Bodyline, Wardrobe, Color, Hair, Make-Up.* Ed. Phyllis Avedon. Los Altos, Calif.: Crisp Publications, 1997.

The Reader's Digest Complete Guide to Sewing. Pleasantville, N.Y.: Reader's Digest Association, Inc., 1976.

Repinski, Karyn, ed. *The Complete Idiot's Guide to Successful Dressing.* New York: Macmillan, 1999.

Saunders, Jan. *Wardrobe Quick-Fixes.* Radnor, Pa.: Chilton Book Company, 1995.

Sulvavik, Christopher, Josh Karlen, and Josh Taylor. *The Indispensable Guide to Classic Men's Clothing.* Brooklyn, N.Y.: Tatra Press, 1999.

Well, Christa. *Secondhand Chic: The Secrets of Finding Fantastic Bargains at Thrift Shops, Consignment Shops, Vintage Shops and More.* New York: Pocket Books, 1999.

Gwen Ellis has worked in publishing for many years, most recently as acquisitions editor for ZonderKidz. She is the author of *Decorating on a Shoestring, The Big Book of Family Fun,* and ten other books. She is a motivational speaker and can hold workshops for your group on *Dress like a Million Bucks without Spending It!* or *Decorating on a Shoestring.*

Jo Ann Janssen is a writer and homemaker in Colorado Springs, Colorado, and the author of *Decorating on a Shoestring.*